171
712
19.9.19

AF654847

Anthropology in Public Health

By Prof. Subir Biswas

- Anthropology and Tribal Development
- Ethical Issues in Anthropological Research
- Human Health: A Bio-Cultural Synthesis

About the Editors

Mithun Das is an Assistant Professor in Anthropology and Head, Department of Anthropology at Sree Chaitanya College, Habra, West Bengal, India. He was awarded the Raman Post-Doctoral Fellowship 2014-15 to study in USA from the University Grants Commission, New Delhi, India. He worked as Visiting Scientist at the University of Alabama at Birmingham, USA, Department of Epidemiology, School of Public Health under the mentorship of Prof. Donna K. Arnett on Epigenetics of Metabolic Syndrome and related phenotypes. His current interests include genetic, epigenetic and lifestyle factors related to ethnic variations in susceptibility to complex diseases like cardiovascular diseases, hypertension, type 2 diabetes and metabolic syndrome. Till date he has over 20 publications in several peer reviewed journals like *PLoS One, Frontiers in Genetics, Journal of Nutrition Health and Ageing, Diabetes Research and Clinical Practice, Journal of Cardiovascular Disease Research, Human Biology, American Journal of Human Biology, Anthropologischer Anzeiger,* and *Collegium Antropologicum.*

Subir Biswas is Professor and former Head, Department of Anthropology, West Bengal State University, Barasat, Kolkata. Earlier he was an Assistant Professor at Department of Anthropology of North Bengal University (since 2001). His area of interests are Anthropological demography, Gender, Health and Bioethics. He has to his credit several research projects of UGC, ICSSR, CWS (NBU), UGC-IUC associateship at IIAS, Shimla; and successfully guided five doctorate scholars. He has published five edited books as well as several research articles of anthropological interests published in national and international journals.

Anthropology in Public Health

Edited by

Mithun Das
Subir Biswas

CONCEPT PUBLISHING COMPANY PVT. LTD.
NEW DELHI-110059

© Editors

All rights reserved. No part of this work may be reproduced, stored, adapted, or transmitted in any form or by any means, electronic, mechanical, photocopying, micro-filming recording or otherwise, or translated in any language, without the prior written permission of the copyright owner and the publisher. The book is sold subject to the condition that it shall not, by way of trade or otherwise, be lent, resold, hired out, or otherwise circulated without the prior publisher's written consent in any form of binding or cover other than that in which it is published.

The views and opinions expressed in this book are author(s) own and the facts reported by him/her have been verified to the extent possible, and the publishers are not in any way liable for the same.

ISBN-13: 978-93-86682-87-1

First Published 2019

Published and Printed by

Concept Publishing Company Pvt. Ltd.
A/15-16, Commercial Block, Mohan Garden,
New Delhi-110059 (INDIA)
T: +91 11 25351460, +91 11 25351794
E : publishing@conceptpub.com, *W* : www.conceptpub.com

Cataloging in Publication Data--Courtesy: D.K. Agencies (P) Ltd. <docinfo@dkagencies.com>

National Seminar on "Role of Anthropology in Public Health" (2017 : Habra, India)
Anthropology in public health / edited by Mithun Das, Subir Biswas.
pages cm
Contributed articles.
"... Anthropological Survey of India, Kolkata and Indian Council of Medical Research, New Delhi for sponsoring the National Seminar on "Role of Anthropology in Public Health" held on 18-19 March, 2017 at Sree Chaitanya College, Habra, West Bengal"—Page viii.
Includes bibliographical references and index.
ISBN 9789386682871

1. Tribes—Medical care—India, Northeastern—Congresses. 2. Chronic diseases—India, Northeastern—Congresses. 3. Tribes—Nutrition—India, Northeastern—Congresses. 4. Tribes—Health and hygiene—India, Northeastern—Congresses. 5. Public health—Anthropological aspects—India, Northeastern—Congresses. I. Das, Mithun, editor. II. Biswas, Subir, 1974- editor. III. Sree Chaitanya College (Habra, India), host institution. IV. Anthropological Survey of India, sponsoring body. V. Indian Council of Medical Research, sponsoring body. VI. Title.

LCC RA529.N38 2017 | DDC 362.109541 23

Foreword

Anthropology, by definition, is the study of man. It does so by investigating both social and biological aspects of human variation and evolution. It deals with human populations. On the other hand, public health encompasses the investigation of factors associated with health of populations. Therein lies the confluence of anthropology and public health, i.e. the study of various factors associated with diseases in human populations.

This book titled *Anthropology in Public Health* explores the relationship of some important factors involved in the causation (as well as responses to) of both communicable and non-communicable diseases in various Indian populations. It deals with the biological and social determinants of these ailments. The book also investigates not only the awareness of these diseases but also the health seeking behaviours. In general, the emphasis of this book is the role anthropology plays in public health. This is highlighted with special reference to particular diseases.

In total, there are fifteen very well written and lucid chapters by various researchers from different institutions of East and North-East India. It is noteworthy, that this book will be very useful not only for students and researchers of anthropology, public health, epidemiology, medicine, but, also for all other professionals who are interested in the study of morbidity in Indian populations.

I congratulate the editors for their commendable effort. I look forward to more such publications from them in future.

Prof. Kaushik Bose,
D.Sc.

Preface

Looking backward over the last few decades, it is impressive to see how far anthropological approaches to public health have come up, not just on communicable disease research and prevention, but also for non-communicable diseases like cardiovascular diseases, diabetes, cancer, female reproductive health, mental illness, substance consumption and abuse, and health practices. Yet, when countries with established economy are compared with low economy countries, there seem to be a radical difference. Anthropologists with their extensive fieldwork and vast well grounded theoretical knowledge plays a significant role in public health arena.

One of the most attractive features of this book is that the editors have asked the authors to lay out the specific methods of their research projects and programmes, so, that the reader can come to a sense of where this field is going. We envision the audience of this book to comprise a broad spectrum of those involved in anthropology, public health and epidemiology. The readers will find this book presenting a familiar public health milieu in a different and fascinating context. Individuals who are just beginners in these fields will find these chapters foundational in careers.

The first part of the book comprises three chapters related to *Health Care Practices and Awareness*. Here, we begin with existential consequences of explanatory models and health seeking behaviour through contrasting case studies of Santals and Drukpas of West Bengal. Next chapter attempts to put anthropological insights of health awareness among the Kandha of Odisha. Third chapter shows the challenges of health care and sanitation among the Birhor of Hazaribag, Jharkhand.

The second part of the book is comprised four chapters (chapters 4-7) devoted to *Epidemiology of Non-Communicable Disease*. Chapter 4 gives interesting insight into the social determinants of

Cardiovascular Diseases. The next chapter gives valuable knowledge on the effect of family history of disease and metabolic risk factors on diabetes phenotype among the people living in and around Kolkata. Chapter 6 is a review of epidemiology of hypothyroidism in North East Indian population. The second part of the books ends with the incidence of type 2 diabetes among the physically active and inactive population of Manipur.

The third part of the book is comprised four chapters (chapters 8-11) related to *Fertility and Mortality*. This part begins with fertility and mortality profile among the Khasi of Meghalaya. Next chapter puts emphasis on anthropological analysis of infant mortality among the tribes of Krushnanagar in Khorda, Odisha. This is followed by a study on differential fertility and mortality among the Vadabalija women of Visakhapatnam, Andhra Pradesh. The last chapter of this part is a study on segregation and distortion of ABO and Rh blood groups and reproductive performance in Bengali population.

The fourth and last part of the book is also comprised four chapters (chapters 12-15) devoted to *Nutritional Status*. This part begins with overweight and socio-economic conditions among adult Meitei males of Manipur. Next chapter shows correlation between socio-economic status and body mass index among the Khond of Andhra Pradesh. Chapter 14 is very interesting as well as informative. It shows the nutritional status of the hand rickshaw pullers of Kolkata. The last chapter shows the prevalence of malnutrition among male and female of Annavaram village in Visakhapatnam, Andhra Pradesh.

The editors are thankful to Anthropological Survey of India, Kolkata and Indian Council of Medical Research, New Delhi for sponsoring the National Seminar on "Role of Anthropology in Public Health" held on 18-19 March, 2017 at Sree Chaitanya College, Habra, West Bengal. Some selected papers presented in the seminar were asked for contributing to make this edited volume.

We are thankful and oblige to Prof. Basab Chaudhuri, Hon'ble Vice Chancellor of West Bengal State University as being our Chief Patron and Dr. Indramohan Mandal, Principal, Sree Chaitanya College, Habra, West Bengal, as being President of the Seminar; as well as to our organizing committee members for making the seminar a grand success.

We never claim that we have been able to do justice to all the areas involved in the present work, but honestly, we tried to give our best effort to satisfy the least to the readers.

We would like to sincerely thank the chapter authors for taking time from their busy schedule to create, what we believe, is a truly engaging and useful book. Their expertise and insights have not only been a gift to us, we hope, it will be gift to all interested readers as well.

Mithun Das
Subir Biswas

Contents

PART-III

Fertility and Mortality

PART-IV

Nutritional Status

Public Health: A Note

Subho Roy

Health and well-being is a matter of concern to all strata of the society. It is a tall order to envision a society which is free from the perennial struggle against diseases.

A concern for health is one thing we can share in common. We all have experiences of diseases and disability throughout our lives and a particular state of health allows individuals to participate in society. In public health, personal health is seen in relation to community health. For example, a measure of success of national public health includes life expectancy tables. So, public health is a collective response to threats against people's health. Its academic interest lies not only in the understanding of the relationship between health and society, but may go beyond in advocacy and policy development. Public health initiatives involve collective action or treatments that affect the population, because it is thoroughly social and political enterprise. A myriad of academic disciplines, like Anthropology, Sociology, Psychology, Demography, Human Genetics and Human Physiology are working independently or in collaboration to enrich the body of knowledge of public health.

While the concept of "old public health" was restricted to health protection and disease prevention, the "new public health" adds the dimensions of health promotion and health development. Studies in public health started with the sanitation movement in the nineteenth century focusing on infectious diseases. Later, in the mid of the twentieth century emphasis was laid on risk factor epidemiology. Social epidemiology became an important component of studying public health during the later part of the twentieth century. The researchers in the area of public health draw upon a variety of frameworks, which ranges from biomedical and lifestyle to feminist, political economy, human rights and eco-social framework.

Anthropology as a discipline understands public health problems within a larger ecological/evolutionary, social, cultural, historical and political context. For example, Anthropologists may take a bio-cultural approach in looking into the issue of public health problems—as an interaction among the human biology, ecology and culture. Or, they may contextualize the public health problems from the perspective of the people under study. Thus, they generate a rich body of knowledge concerning the attitude and practices surrounding health of a community; social organization and norms that affect care-giving; and the "local moral world" including local religious norms, that surround the therapeutic decision-making and the acceptance/rejection of public health innovations. Some also argue that economic organization and relationship of power are the principal forces determining human sickness and health. These are imperative at the conceptualization stage of policy development to initiate any intervention programme. Anthropologists also take the role of a critique to public health policies. The theory of neo-liberalism, which focuses on the privatization of public health and biomedical services around the globe, is critically assessed. Some scholars also argue that public health from the Durkeimian concept of the cult of humanity. It argues that public health has now partially filled the gap left in contemporary society created in the decline of religion and the rise of cult of humanity. It further argues that if religious belief declined then other belief systems would be need to maintain cohesive forces for secular industrial society. In other words, public health has extended from its scientific foundation to have a wider role as a moral force influencing international and national health policies around the world and even mediating between different institutions, including the state and the market.

List of Contributors

Arnab Ghosh, Dr., Assistant Professor, Department of Anthropology, Visva Bharati, Santiniketan-731235, Birbhum, West Bengal. E-mail: *arnab_cu@rediffmail.com*

Arup Ratan Bandyopadhyay, Professor, Department of Anthropology, University of Calcutta, Kolkata-700019. E-mail: *arup.cu@gmail.com*

Diptendu Chatterjee, Dr. Assistant Professor, Department of Anthropology, University of Calcutta, Kolkata-700019. E-mail: *dip_cu@rediffmail.com*

Divya Bharti, Research Scholar, Anthropological Survey of India, Central Regional Centre, Nagpur-440006, Maharashtra. E-mail: *divyamehta.mehta104@gmail.com*

Duka Devi Chhetri, Research scholar, Department of Anthropology, Sikkim University, Tadong-737102, Sikkim. E-mail: *raniduka92@gmail.com*

Ganga Nath Jha, Dr. Assistant Professor, Department of Anthropology, Vinoba Bhave University, Hazaribag-825301, Jharkhand. E-mail: *gangajharkhand@gmail.com*

Indrani Lodh, Dr. Director, Urvaraa IVF Clinic, 40/1a, 1st floor, Hazra Road, Ballygunge, Kolkata-700019, West Bengal. E-mail: *drindranilodh@yahoo.co.*

Jibananda Gayen, Dr. Assistant Professor, Department of Geography, Sree Chaitanya College, Habra, North 24 Parganas-743268, West Bengal. E-mail: *jibananda07@gmail.com*

Kaushik Bose, Professor, Department of Anthropology, Vidyasagar University, Midnapore-721102, West Bengal. E-mail: *kaushikbose@cantab.net*

Kh Dimkhohoi Baite, Research Scholar, Department of Anthropology, Manipur University, Imphal-795003, Manipur. E-mail: *didimbaite@gmail.com*

Ksh. BeliyaLuxmi Devi, Research Scholar, Department of Anthropology, Manipur University, Imphal-795003, Manipur. E-mail: *beliya.kshetri@yahoo.in*

Maibam Samson Singh, Dr. Assistant Professor, Department of Anthropology, Sikkim University, Tadong-737102, Sikkim. E-mail: *mssingh@cus.ac.in*

Mithun Das, Dr. Assistant Professor, Department of Anthropology, Sree Chaitanya College, Habra, North 24 Parganas-743268. West Bengal. E-mail: *mithundas01@yahoo.com*

Mong Fing Lepcha, Research Scholar, Department of Anthropology, Sikkim University, Tadong-737102, Sikkim. E-mail: *mongfingemail@gmail.com*

Moumita Sadhukhan, Research Scholar, Department of Anthropology, University of Calcutta, Kolkata-700019, West Bengal. E-mail: *sadhukhan.sarmili@gmail.com*

Paramananda Naik, Research Scholar, P.G. Department of Anthropology, Utkal University, Khorda-751004, Odisha. E-mail: *paramananda090@gmail.com*

Pinak Tarafdar, Dr. Assistant Professor, Department of Anthropology, University of North Bengal, Darjeeling-734013, West Bengal. E-mail: *pinaknbu@gmail.com*

Pranab Kr. Das, Dr. Assistant Professor, Department of Geography, Sree Chaitanya College, Habra, North 24 Parganas-743268, West Bengal. E-mail: *pranabtaki@gmail.com*

Pranabesh Sarkar, Research Scholar, Department of Anthropology, University of Calcutta, Kolkata-700019, West Bengal. E-mail: *p.sarkar1991@gmail.com*

Riddhi Goswami, Dr. Assistant Professor, Department of Biotechnology, Heritage Institute of Technology, Kolkata-700107, West Bengal. E-mail: *riddhigoswami@heritageit.edu*

S. Jibonkumar Singh, Dr. Professor, Department of Anthropology, Manipur University, Imphal-795003, Manipur. E-mail: *drjibonkumar@yahoo.com*

S. Yaiphaba Meitei, Dr. Assistant Professor, Department of Anthropology, Manipur University, Imphal-795003, Manipur. E-mail: *yaipha_meitei@yahoo.co.in*

Sagar Chettri, Dr. Assistant Professor, Department of Anthropology, Sikkim University, Tadong-737102, Sikkim. E-mail: *zenithc6@gmail.com*

Sanghamitra Sethi, Research Scholar, P.G. Department of Anthropology, Utkal University, Khorda-751004, Odisha. E-mail: *ssmitra048@gmail.com*

Subho Roy, Professor, Department of Anthropology, University of Calcutta, Kolkata-700019, West Bengal. E-mail: *subharay@rediffmail.com*

Subir Biswas, Professor and Former Head, Department of Anthropology, West Bengal State University, Barasat, Kolkata, West Bengal. E-mail: *gargisubir@gmail.com*

Part-I

Health Care Practices and Awareness

1

Explanatory Models and Health Seeking Behaviour

The Existential Consequences

Pinak Tarafdar

Introduction

The pivotal task of a medical anthropologist is to explore the explanatory models of individuals suffering by any kind of ailments or related misfortunes. It is a personal elucidation of etiology, treatment, and outcome of sickness by which a patient, family member and healers explain the entire phenomena. Hence, Explanatory models are the learned cultural models and subsequently shared by an ethnic community.

Explanatory Model

In the context of medical pluralism, clinicians can elicit the person's explanatory model of his or her sickness rather than memorize the details of specific ethnomedical belief system (Brown *et al.*, 1997). An explanatory model is a personal interpretation of the etiology, treatment and outcome of sickness by which person gives meaning to his or her condition. Although EMs is personal, they are also learned cultural models, so, that an EM shared by a group might be considered a folk model of disease. These models constitute health belief systems that, from cross-cultural perspective, generally fall into two categories:

1. *Personalistic belief systems*: that explain sickness as the result of supernatural forces directed at a patient, either by a sorcerer or by an angry sprit; and

2. *Naturalistic belief systems*: that explain sickness in terms of natural forces, such as the germ theory of contagion in Western biomedicine.

Klienman's in his article "Culture, Illness and Care" examines explanatory model in a clinical setting and also elucidates the reflection of such models in terms of social class, cultural belief, religious affiliation and past experience with health care. Being a medical practitioner it was convenient for him to conduct the research in a clinical setting. Afterwards the same models have been explored by other Anthropologists in different social settings and eventually developed a comprehensive definition of explanatory model (Brown *et al.*, 1997). It is crucial to recognise that patient-doctor interactions are transactions between explanatory models, transactions often involving major discrepancies in cognitive content as well as therapeutic values, expectations and goals (Freidson, 1961; King, 1962).

Moreover, there are three structural domains of health care in society: professional; popular (family, social network, community); and folk (non-professional healers) as mentioned by Kleinman (1973). Each domain possesses its own explanatory systems, social roles, interaction setting, and institutions (Kleinman, 1975). For example, a sufferer is a sick family member or friend in the popular domain, a specific type of patient in the professional domain, and a client of one sort or another in the folk domain. These roles can be quite distinct.

Health Seeking Behaviour: It refers to the process whereby people seek medical assistance and select health care practitioners. It has also been defined as any action undertaken by individuals who perceive themselves to have a health problem or to be ill for the purpose of finding an appropriate remedy (Ward, Mertens and Thomas, 1997). The explanatory model of a particular illness consists of signs and symptoms by which the illness is recognised; presumed cause of the illness and prognosis established (Foster and Anderson, 1978; and Kleinman, 1980).

The Present Discourse: The present discourse is intended to unfold a critical appraisal whether explanatory models are alone good predictors of people's observed pattern of health seeking? OR The various factors like influence of family members, socio-economic condition, gender variations, communication and access to health resources may affect the said decision-making process.

Seeking of medical assistance and choosing of health care practitioners may also be seemingly understood as categories of treatments and more fundamentally the same is categorised as traditional and modern or biomedical treatment. In the present context I concentrate primarily on explanatory models of patients or the close accompanies in connection with the cause of ailments.

Study 1

Three distinctive types of Santal villages were selected considering the scope and objectives of the study. The 'type' explains the criteria, viz. distance from the sub-divisional town (Jhargram), as well as sub-divisional hospital, communication, biomedical health facilities surrounding the villages. The fieldwork for the study has been conducted during 2002-2005.

Category of Villages

'Type' One villages are longest in distance from the urban centre and health facility is negligible in comparison with the other two 'types'. No primary health centre or sub-centre is situated in a short distance. Very ill-equipped communication to any of the urban/semi-urban places. The absence of quack and private doctor in a shortest distance is another additional criterion. In case of 'Type' Two villages the distance from the urban centre/hospital is longer than 'type' three, but shorter than 'type' one. Further, a rural hospital, some private doctors and quacks are available in close vicinity. Moreover, the villages are also well communicated to the sub-divisional hospital. The Type Three villages are closest to the urban centre with the contemporary biomedical health care facilities, viz. hospital, nursing home, private practitioner, diagnostic centres etc. But the road communication system is not up to the mark like 'type' two villages.

Results and Discussion

Explanatory models of the male patients are more inclined towards naturalistic cause of disease causation. The number increases as it proceeds from type-1 to type-3 villages more elaborately from distant to nearby urban centre (Table 1.1). Surprisingly females have opined just the antagonistic views as most of them from type-2 villages suffered by female diseases (Table 1.2). In spite of a rural hospital adjacent village, the villagers of Shalukdoba tried to explain the reason of irregular menstrual cycle as a direct consequence of ghost attack. On the other hand villagers of Valuka another 'type'-two village and one of the highest literate populations under the study are in denial of any such incidence.

Table 1.1: Causes of Ailments (Male, Study-1)

Village Type	*Villages*	*Tribe*	*Male*			
			Natural	*Superna-tural*	*Unknown*	*Total*
ONE	Agaya	Santal	02 (11.76)	03 (17.64)	12 (70.58)	17 (100.00)
		Kora	—	02 (66.67)	01 (33.33)	03 (100.00)
	Total		02 (10.00)	05 (25.00)	13 (65.00)	20 (100.00)
	Barashyamnagar	Santal	05 (27.77)	03 (16.66)	10 (55.55)	18 (100.00)
TOTAL			**07 (18.42)**	**08 (21.05)**	**23 (60.53)**	**38 (100.00)**
TWO	Shalukdoba	Santal	10 (41.66)	04 (16.66)	10 (41.66)	24 (100.00)
	Valuka	Santal	01 (20.00)	02 (40.00)	02 (40.00)	05 (100.00)
TOTAL			**11 (37.93)**	**06 (20.69)**	**12 (41.38)**	**29 (100.00)**
THREE	Laredi	Santal	13 (44.82)	08 (27.59)	08 (27.59)	29 (100.00)
	Kutusgeria	Santal	06 (37.5)	02 (12.5)	08 (50.00)	16 (100.00)
TOTAL			**19 (42.22)**	**10 (22.22)**	**16 (35.56)**	**45 (100.00)**
GRAND TOTAL			**37 (33.03)**	**24 (21.43)**	**51 (45.54)**	**112 (100.00)**

Note: Figures in brackets showing percentages.
Source: Tarafdar, 2005.

Table 1.2: Causes of Ailments (Female, Study-1)

Village Type	*Villages*	*Tribe*	*Female*			
			Natural	*Superna-tural*	*Unknown*	*Total*
ONE	Agaya	Santal	07 (63.63)	01 (9.09)	03 (27.27)	11 (100.00)
		Kora	01 (16.66)	03 (50.00)	02 (33.33)	06 (100.00)
	Total		08 (47.06)	04 (23.53)	05 (29.41)	17 (100.00)
	Barashyamnagar	Santal	02 (11.11)	05 (27.77)	11 (61.11)	18 (100.00)
TOTAL			**10 (28.57)**	**09 (25.71)**	**16 (45.71)**	**35 (100.00)**
TWO	Shalukdoba	Santal	06 (20.68)	08 (27.58)	15 (51.72)	29 (100.00)
	Valuka	Santal	04 (44.44)	02 (22.22)	03 (33.33)	09 (100.00)
TOTAL			**10 (26.32)**	**10 (26.32)**	**18 (47.37)**	**38 (100.00)**
THREE	Laredi	Santal	04 (23.53)	03 (17.65)	10 (58.52)	17 (100.00)
	Kutusgeria	Santal	02 (28.57)	02 (28.57)	03 (42.86)	07 (100.00)
TOTAL			**06 (25.00)**	**05 (20.83)**	**13 (54.17)**	**24 (100.00)**
GRAND TOTAL			**26 (26.8)**	**24 (24.74)**	**47 (48.45)**	**97 (100.00)**

Note: Figures in brackets showing percentages.
Source: Tarafdar, 2005.

Results and Discussion

In the present study low percentage of availing traditional treatment has much shaped by the unavailability and decreasing efficiency of the healers and less-tolerance of the patients. They generally avail traditional treatment, in case cause of ailment is identified as supernatural (Tables 1.3 and 1.4).

Santals' visit the traditional healers because of their typical approach and attitude as both of the care giver and receivers share the identical cultural milieu. Santals have the knowledge whether to undergo traditional or biomedical treatments considering the nature of ailments in various situations. But deviation from the usual choice

Table 1.3: Categories of Treatments (Male, Study-1)

Village Type	*Villages*	*Tribe*	*Male*				
			Traditional	*Modern/ Bio-medical*	*Both*	*No*	*Total*
ONE	Agaya	Santal	03 (17.64)	11 (64.7)	03 (17.64)	—	17 (100.00)
		Kora	01 (33.33)	02 (66.66)	—	—	03 (100.00)
	Total		04 (20.00)	13 (65.00)	03 (15.00)	—	20 (100.00)
	Barashyamnagar	Santal	05 (27.77)	10 (55.55)	02 (11.11)	01 (4.16)	18 (100.00)
TOTAL			**09 (23.68)**	**23 (60.53)**	**05 (13.16)**	**01 (2.63)**	**38 (100.00)**
TWO	Shalukdoba	Santal	01 (4.16)	18 (75.00)	04 (16.66)	01 (4.16)	24 (100.00)
	Valuka	Santal	01 (20.00)	02 (40.00)	02 (40.00)	—	05 (100.00)
TOTAL			**02 (6.89)**	**20 (68.97)**	**06 (20.69)**	**01 (3.45)**	**29 (100.00)**
THREE	Laredi	Santal	03 (10.34)	19 (65.52)	07 (24.14)	—	29 (100.00)
	Kutusgeria	Santal	—	14 (87.50)	01 (6.25)	01 (6.25)	16 (100.00)
TOTAL			**03 (6.67)**	**33 (73.33)**	**08 (17.78)**	**01 (2.22)**	**45 (100.00)**
GRAND TOTAL			**14 (12.5)**	**76 (67.85)**	**19 (16.96)**	**03 (2.67)**	**112 (100.00)**

Note: Figures in brackets showing percentages.
Source: Tarafdar, 2005

is also noticed. Further, simultaneously they continue both (traditional and biomedical) treatments in various cases, but some extent not satisfied with any of them due to less availability and more time consuming in the former and not getting the required medicines and infrastructure in the latter.

An overlapping of traditional belief and practices with biomedical system create more confusion among them. Despite of government initiatives poor economic condition and ill communication facilities are the main constraints for not utilizing the biomedical treatment.

Table 1.4: Categories of Treatments (Female, Study-1)

Village Type	*Villages*	*Tribe*	*Female*				
			Traditional	*Modern/ Bio-medical*	*Both*	*No*	*Total*
ONE	Agaya	Santal	03 (27.27)	07 (63.63)	01 (9.09)	—	11 (100.00)
		Kora	01 (16.66)	04 (66.66)	—	01 (16.66)	06 (100.00)
	Total		04 (23.53)	11 (64.71)	01 (5.88)	01 (5.88)	17 (100.00)
	Barashyamnagar	Santal	05 (27.77)	08 (44.44)	05 (27.77)	—	18 (100.00)
TOTAL			**09 (25.71)**	**19 (54.26)**	**06 (17.14)**	**01 (2.86)**	**35 (100.00)**
TWO	Shalukdoba	Santal	06 (20.68)	20 (68.96)	03 (16.34)	—	29 (100.00)
	Valuka	Santal	01 (11.11)	08 (88.89)	—	—	09 (100.00)
TOTAL			**07 (18.42)**	**28 (73.68)**	**09 (23.68)**	**—**	**38 (100.00)**
THREE	Laredi	Santal	01 (5.88)	10 (58.82)	02 (11.76)	04 (23.53)	17 (100.00)
	Kutusgeria	Santal	—	04 (57.14)	01 (14.29)	02 (28.58)	07 (100.00)
TOTAL			**01 (4.16)**	**14 (58.33)**	**03 (12.5)**	**06 (25.00)**	**24 (100.00)**
GRAND TOTAL			**17 (17.5)**	**61 (62.89)**	**12 (12.37)**	**07 (7.22)**	**97 (100.00)**

Note: Figures in brackets showing percentages.
Source: Tarafdar, 2005.

Even the male-female differentiations are also responsible for not availing the expensive biomedical remedies. Santals reside adjacent to an urban centre certainly does not mean that they can avail better modern medical facilities. In some of the cases far-flung inhabited villagers with good communication can access it in a much better and convenient way.

Study 2

The present study was conducted among the 'Drukpas' of Buxa-Duar region of district Jalpaiguri (erstwhile), West Bengal. The Drukpas are Tibeto-Mongoloid in origin and they mainly inhabit in Bhutan along with some population in Sikkim, Assam, and some part of West Bengal, but the present study is conducted in Buxa-Duar region which is situated in the Kalchini block of Jalpaiguri District, West Bengal. The entire zone is under the 'Buxa Tiger Reserve' Forest Project. Incredible landscape, hilly terrain and significant biodiversity with conspicuous number of flora and fauna are the characteristic feature of the zone. The fieldwork for the same has been done during 2011-2013.

Category of Villages

For the convenience of the study the entire Drukpa villages of Buxa-Duar region are categorized on the basis of various predefined and post-confirmed criteria. The above mentioned eight villages of the entire Buxa-Duar region were categorized into two different categories, i.e. category-1 and category-2. Daragaon, Lalbunglow, Lepchakha and Tashigaon are included under the category-1. These villages have less distance from the nearest health centre as well as motor road. The village roads always accessible even in rainy season. Due to moderate communication throughout the year, the health workers of the Family Planning Association of India (FPAI) regularly visit in these villages. Incidentally, in these four villages exclusive Buddhists were found with some negligible Christian households.

On the other hand category-2 is comprises with another four villages, namely Adma, Chunabhati, Namna and Ochlum. These villages are very much inaccessible due to sinuous hills and dense forest; although some of the villages of the present category have very less distance from nearest motor road and health centre even in comparison with category-1 villages. In rainy season the village road is completely inaccessible, which leads to the irregular reciprocal visit of villagers and medical practitioners such as FPAI workers. In these four villages both the Buddhist and the Christian households were found along with the Christian dominancy in some villages like Namna and Chunabhati.

Results and Discussion

As per the explanatory models the people from category-2 villages have reported on their perception which is significantly more of natural causes behind the onset of ailments whereas villages of category-1 are characterised with more accessibility and less distance from the nearest health centre and motor road; but most of the villagers have reported less belief on natural causes for their sickness. Affiliation with specific religion seems to be responsible for such outcome. Except Daragaon all the villages in category-1 are mainly,

Table 1.5: Causes of Ailments (Male, Study-2)

Cate-gories	*Name of the Villages*	*Male*				
		Natural	*Super-natural*	*Both*	*Unknown*	*Total Affected*
Category-1	Daragaon	03 (50.00)	03 (50.00)	—	—	06 (100.00)
	Lalbunglow	29 (72.50)	04 (10.00)	—	07 (17.50)	40 (100.00)
	Lepchakha	30 (90.91)	—	—	03 09.09	33 (100.00)
	Tashigaon	25 (62.50)	13 (32.50)	—	02 (05.00)	40 (100.00)
	Total	**87 (73.11)**	**20 (16.81)**	**—**	**12 (10.08)**	**119 (100.00)**
Category-2	Adma	28 (96.55)	—	01 (03.45)	—	29 (100.00)
	Chunabhati	48 (85.71)	05 (08.93)	—	03 (05.36)	56 (100.00)
	Namna	06 (85.71)	—	—	01 (14.29)	07 (100.00)
	Ochlum	02 (66.67)	—	—	01 (33.33)	03 (100.00)
	Total	**84 (88.42)**	**05 (05.26)**	**01 (01.05)**	**05 (05.26)**	**95 (100.00)**
Grand Total		**171 (79.91)**	**25 (11.68)**	**01 (00.47)**	**17 (07.94)**	**214 (100.00)**

Note: Figures in brackets showing percentages.
Source: Tarafdar, 2013.

Table 1.6: Causes of Ailments (Female, Study-2)

Categories	*Name of the Villages*	*Female*				
		Natural	*Super-natural*	*Both*	*Unknown*	*Total Affected*
Category-1	Daragaon	02 (66.67)	01 (33.33)	—	—	03 (100.00)
	Lalbunglow	15 (60.00)	04 (16.00)	—	06 (24.00)	25 (100.00)
	Lepchakha	32 (91.43)	—	—	03 (08.57)	35 (100.00)
	Tashigaon	18 (62.07)	09 (31.03)	—	02 (06.90)	29 (100.00)
	Total	**67 (72.83)**	**14 (15.22)**	**—**	**11 (11.96)**	**92 (100.00)**
Category-2	Adma	32 (96.97)	—	—	01 (03.03)	33 (100.00)
	Chunabhati	34 (73.91)	06 (13.04)	01 (02.17)	05 (10.87)	46 (100.00)
	Namna	07 (00.00)	—	—	—	07 (100.00)
	Ochlum	06 (75.00)	01 (12.50)	—	01 (12.50)	08 (100.00)
	Total	**79 (84.04)**	**07 (07.45)**	**01 (01.06)**	**07 (07.45)**	**94 (100.00)**
Grand Total		**146 (78.49)**	**21 (11.29)**	**01 (00.54)**	**18 (09.68)**	**186 (100.00)**

Note: Figures in brackets showing percentages.
Source: Tarafdar, 2013.

comprised with the Buddhist people having a considerable less faith on the natural forces for inception of various ailments (Tables 1.5 and 1.6).

In case of category-2 villages, except Ochlum all the other three are inhabited by majority of Drukpa Christian population who rely more on natural causes behind the occurrences of various diseases and misfortunes. Despite a village of category-2 the villagers of Ochlum have opined considerably less on natural belief regarding the disease causation, presumably because of belonging to Buddhist segment. On the other hand being a Buddhist village of category-1 the inhabitant of Lepchakha have reported the high percentage in favour of natural beliefs due to very close contact with the adjoining so-called mainstream people as tourists. Lepchakha is a very famous tourist spot in the entire region for its magnificent scenic view and for observing Losar, the traditional archery competition of the Drukpa (Table 1.5 and 1.6).

Results and Discussion

The Drukpa population under the study have been experiencing traditional (exclusive), modern/biomedical (exclusive) and both (traditional and biomedical) process of treatment. If exclusiveness of availing traditional treatment is compared between the villagers of category-1 and category-2 than the patients from the latter category

Table 1.7: Category of Treatment (Male, Study-2)

Categories	*Name of the Villages*	*Male*				
		Traditional	*Modern/ Bio-medical*	*Both*	*No Treatment*	*Total*
Category-1	Daragaon	01 (16.67)	04 (66.67)	01 (16.67)	—	06 (100.00)
	Lalbunglow	—	08 (20.00)	27 (67.50)	05 (12.50)	40 (100.00)
	Lepchakha	—	31 (93.94)	02 (06.06)	—	33 (100.00)
	Tashigaon	01 (02.50)	25 (62.50)	13 (32.50)	01 (02.50)	40 (100.00)
	Total	**02 (01.68)**	**68 (57.14)**	**43 (36.13)**	**06 (05.04)**	**119 (100.00)**
Category-2	Adma	01 (03.45)	24 (82.76)	03 (10.34)	01 (03.45)	29 (100.00)
	Chunabhati	05 (08.93)	44 (78.57)	02 (03.57)	05 (08.93)	56 (100.00)
	Namna	—	06 (85.71)	—	01 (14.29)	07 (100.00)
	Ochlum	—	02 (66.67)	01 (33.33)	—	03 (100.00)
	Total	**06 (06.32)**	**76 (80.00)**	**06 (06.32)**	**07 (07.37)**	**95 (100.00)**
Grand Total		**08 (03.74)**	**144 (67.29)**	**49 (22.90)**	**13 (06.07)**	**214 (100.00)**

Note: Figures in brackets showing percentages.
Source: Tarafdar, 2013.

Table 1.8: Category of Treatment (Female, Study-2)

Categories	*Name of the Villages*	*Female*				
		Tradi-tional	*Modern/ Bio-medical*	*Both*	*No Treat-ment*	*Total*
Category-1	Daragaon	—	31 (00.00)	—	—	03 (100.00)
	Lalbunglow	—	02 (08.00)	19 (76.00)	04 (16.00)	25 (100.00)
	Lepchakha	—	31 (88.57)	01 (02.86)	03 (09.09)	35 (100.00)
	Tashigaon	—	19 (65.52)	09 (31.03)	01 (03.45)	29 (100.00)
	Total	**—**	**55 (59.78)**	**29 (31.52)**	**08 (08.70)**	**92 (100.00)**
Category-2	Adma	01 (03.03)	28 (84.85)	—	04 (12.12)	33 (100.00)
	Chunabhati	04 (07.14)	33 (78.57)	04 (08.69)	05 (10.87)	46 (100.00)
	Namna	—	06 (85.71)	—	01 (14.29)	07 (100.00)
	Ochlum	—	07 (87.50)	01 (12.50)	—	08 (100.00)
	Total	**05 (05.32)**	**74 (78.72)**	**05 (05.32)**	**10 (10.64)**	**94 (100.00)**
Grand Total		**05 (02.69)**	**129 (69.35)**	**34 (18.28)**	**18 (09.68)**	**186 (100.00)**

Note: Figures in brackets showing percentages.
Source: Tarafdar, 2013.

have sought more in numbers but surprisingly in case of exclusively availed biomedical treatment the same result demands separate connotation (Tables 1.7 and 1.8).

It can be understood by the fact of availing both (traditional and biomedical) treatment processes conspicuously more among the category-1 villagers. The criteria of village selection undoubtedly signifies little bit closeness to the modern health institutions and better route for accessing the nearest motor roads and these are manifested for the category-1 villages. Subsequently most of the villagers of the category-1 belong to the Buddhist religion and more often accentuated to traditional health care system.

Moreover, for better accessibility the category-1 villages are being more intervening by FPAI members. So, it is really a dichotomy between tradition *verses* modern, rather due to such transitional feature the category-1 villagers significantly avail both (traditional and biomedical) the treatment modalities. On the contrary despite of tedious trekking route and ill communication category-2 villagers' have experienced significantly more biomedical treatment due to impact of Christianity in those villages.

Conclusion

Hence, both of the studies explore the importance of understanding explanatory models for evaluating cultural dimension of health. The present discourse also identifies the connection between explanatory models and Health Seeking Behaviour. While disseminating both of the empirical studies which have been taken place in distinctive situations and on different populations, it is evident that along with explanatory models particularly connected with disease causation, the influence of family members, socio-economic condition, gender variations, communication and access to health resources (both traditional and biomedical) also govern the health seeking behaviour. Furthermore, religious affiliation is an additional criterion in this regard.

References

Brown, Peter J., J. Gregg and B. Ballard (1997). "Culture, ethnicity and the practice of medicine", In: Alan Stoudemire (ed.) *Human Behaviour for Medical Students*, New York: Lippincott.

Foster, G.M. and B.G. Anderson (1978). *Medical Anthropology*, New York: John Wiley & Sons.

Freidson, E. (1961). *Patients' Views of Medical Practice,* New York: Russell Sage Foundation.

King, S. (1962). *Perception of Illness in Medical Practice*, New York: Russell Sage Foundation.

Kleinman, A.M. (1973). "Toward a comparative study of medical system", *Science, Medicine, Man,* 1: 55-65.

Kleinman, A.M. (1975). "Explanatory models in health care relationships", *Health of the Family,* Washington D.C.: National Council International Health Symposium, pp. 159-172.

Kleinman, A. (1980). *Patients and Healers in the Context of Culture: An Exploration of the Borderland between Anthropology, Medicine, and Psychiatry,* Berkeley: University of California Press.

Tarafdar, P. (2005). *Concept of Health, Disease and Treatment in the Selected Tribal Villages of Jhargram Sub-division, District-Midnapore, West Bengal,* Unpublished Ph.D. Thesis, University of Calcutta, Kolkata.

Tarafdar, P. (2013). *Health Seeking Behaviour among the Drukpa's of Buxa-Duar Region, District Jalpaiguri, West Bengal,* Unpublished Project Report submitted to ICSSR.

Ward, H., Mertens, T. and Thomas, C. (1997). "Health seeking behaviour and the control of sexually transmitted disease", *Health Policy and Planning,* 12: 19-28.

2

Anthropological Insights of Health Awareness among Kandha in Rayagada District, Odisha

Paramananda Naik

Introduction

Health is a positive state of well-being in which harmonious development of physical and mental capacities of individual lead to enjoyment of rich and full life. Health is thus vital for concurrent and integrated development of the individual and community and for socio-economic development of the country. "Health as a state of complete physical, mental, and social well-being and not merely the absence of disease and infirmity" (WHO, 1971). Health is the one of the most important aspects of human life. The Millennium Development Goals (MDGs) has also emphasized "Health for all". The National Health Mission (NHM) encompasses its two sub-missions, the National Rural Health Mission (NRHM) and National Urban Health Mission (NUHM). The National Health Mission (NHM) envisages achievement of universal access to equitable, affordable and quality health care services that are accountable and responsive to people's needs. As per the Twelfth Five Year Plan document of the Planning Commission, the flagship programme of NRHM will be strengthened under the umbrella of National Health Mission. National Rural Health Mission (NRHM) was launched in April 2005 with a commitment to provide effective health care to the rural population throughout the country with special focus on 18 low performing States including Odisha. National Urban Health Mission (NUHM) was launched in May 2013 with the health concerns of the urban poor population. Health of indigenous or tribal people is the perception and conception in their own cultural system with less awareness of the modern health care and health sources.

Various international declarations, the constitutional guidelines and the Supreme Court judgements are in favour of Right to Health and Health Care. Various UN health rights instruments refer to health related Rights. Though the Constitution of India has not included the right to health care as a Constitutional Right, the Supreme Court in its judgements has interpreted Article 21 (Fundamental Right to Life) and Article 47 of the Directive Principles (which mentions improving health of the citizens as one of the duties of the Government) to mean the right to life as right to life with dignity, including access to basic health care as a right (Phadke, 2003). Since a majority of the Indian population lives in rural areas, variations in the performances of rural health systems get reflected in the overall health outcomes of different States. Central to the rural health systems in India is the primary health centre, established and managed by the public sector. In the Constitution of India, the public provision of health care is a responsibility shared by the Central State, and Local Governments, although it is effectively a State responsibility in terms of delivery. State and local governments account for about three-quarters and the Centre for about a quarter of public spending on health, though there are large variations across States (Sankar and Kathuria, 2004). The theoretical channels from improved health to better education vary in nature over the course of an individual's life. Good health can alter the population growth rate in ways that promote development. Health improvements have the greatest effect on the most vulnerable, children in particular (Bloom, 2005). Health equity is a multi-dimensional concept that involves not only increasing access to healthcare, but also to improving the conditions in which people live and work, influencing their opportunities to be in good health or the social determinants of health. Health equity refers to the absence of systematic differences in health and opportunities in health between social groups that are unfair, avoidable and amenable to intervention (Mohindra *et al.*, 2012). The primary health care infrastructure provides the first level of contact between the population and health care providers. In rural primary health care infrastructure divided into three sub-divisions, such as Sub-Centre, Primary Health Centre

(PHC) and Community Health Centre (CHC). Health promotion is very relevant today. Health or ill health is the result of a combination of different factors. There are different perspectives in expressing the determinants of health of an individual or a community. Holistic health concepts are four major determinants of health or ill health, such as human biology, environment, behaviour and health care organization. As on 1st March, 2011 India's population stood at 121 crores comprising 62.37 crores (51.54%) males and 58.63 crores (48.46%) females. India, which accounts for world's 17.5 per cent population, is the second most populous country in the world next only to China (19.4%). 121 crore Indians, 83.3 crore (68.84%) live in rural areas while 37.7 crores (31.16%) live in urban areas, as per the Census of India, 2011. Tribal population is found in almost all parts of India and Odisha claims to be the largest leading tribal state after Madhya Pradesh and Maharashtra in the country. Tribal communities constitute 8.6 per cent of India's population. In India 705 tribal groups and including 75 PVTGs (Particularly Vulnerable Tribal Groups) (Census of India, 2011). Odisha is the second largest tribal populated state in India. There are 62 categories of Scheduled Tribes including 13 PVTGs and 93 categories of Scheduled Castes in the State. Out of the 62 tribal groups, Kandha are the most populous tribe with a population of 13,95,643 constituting 17.1 per cent of the total Scheduled Tribe (ST) population. The background of this research tends to discover the truth of reality about Kandha people and health awareness among them. The Kandha tribe of India has a typical tribal life style. Basic needs are fulfilled by forest trees and plants. The tribe is also engaged in fishing and cultivation. Among all researches anthropological research towards Man and his related environment in a holistic sphere is something unique. The basic proposition of holism in anthropology is that human behaviour and human health arises out of complex interactions taking place within the cultural systems (Haviland, 2008: 34). Anthropological investigations believed more on micro-studies as human realities become the central focus. So, diagnostic studies provide more achievable knowledge about the limited society, aims to generalize on a macro-level. Mahapatra (1994), therefore, sees health among tribal groups as a functional and not clinical concept. Sachchidananda (1994) sees the field of tribal health aspects as a cultural concept as well as a part of social structure and organization which is continuously changing and adapting itself to changes in the wider society. Singh (1994) indicates nine factors to examine and assess the tribal health situation in India. He highlights the effect of changing physical environment on tribal health, which is ultimately related to their economic pursuits, nutritional, availability, medicines etc. It has also been emphasized that ecology and tribal health is intimately related. Guite and Acharya (2006) have shown that the acceptance of a particular health care system among the tribal people mostly depends on its availability and accessibility. It is interesting to note that while the tribal groups following traditional religion traditional medicines putting religious or supernatural value on it, the converted Christian tribes use the some medicine excluding its religious tribal society is understood not as phenomena in isolation. Tribal health is closely related to culture, environment and the social structure as can be observed from the cultural and medical system. Health in a tribal society in understood not as phenomena in isolation, but in relation to the magico-religious fabric of existence. Tribal health has also to be understood from the context of it being placed in the modern world with all its modernity and the tribal concepts and understanding of their health related to practices and beliefs.

Study Area and People

According to the 2011 Census Rayagada district has a population of 9,61,959. The district has a predominant tribal population of 57.52 per cent. This district has eleven blocks covered under tribal sub-plan with three micro-projects in operation for the pre-literate indigenous tribal communities. The topography of Rayagada gives a perfect platform for the tribal's in sustaining their ethno-cultural identity in the district. The population of Kandha in Odisha is 16.27 lakh as per 2011 Census. The word 'Kandha' is derived from the Telugu word "Konda", which means a small hill as well as the hill men. Kandha a small *adivasi* community people who reside in the Eastern Ghats of Odisha, India. Kandha speaks "Kui" language, a Dravidian linguistic group. On the basis of socio-cultural characteristics, the Kandha may be divided into several sections, such as Desia Kandha, Dongria Kandha, Kutia Kandha, Sitha Kandha, Buda Kandha, Pengo Kandha and Malua Kandha (Table 2.1).

Table 2.1: Rural Health Care System in Rayagada

Sl. No.	*Centre*	*Population Basis in Plain Area*	*Population Basis in Hilly/Tribal/Difficult Terrain Area*
1.	Sub-Centre	5,000	3,000
2.	Primary Health Centre	30,000	20,000
3.	Community Health Centre	1,20,000	80,000

Source: CDMO, Rayagada.

Materials and Methods

The study is based on the assumption that perception of health and health awareness among Kandha people, which in turns influence the health seeking behaviour among people. The study is based on fieldwork. The study has been conducted in Rayagada block of Odisha state. Cluster Random Sampling and Purposive Sampling are used for collection of data from the respondent. This Chapter is based on qualitative study conducted using of primary data collection was In-depth interview and Focus Group Discussions (FGDs). Secondary Information has been collected from various documents such as books, magazines, journals and old research papers as well as from internet etc. The population is about 620 out of which 155 households. Eight focus group discussions with the health worker in three different villages and total of 134 participants were included in the study using in-depth interview and focus group discussions.

Results

The purpose of the study to review the effectiveness on health awareness among Kandha people of Odisha. It thus, discussed empirical documentations on Information, Education and Communication (IEC) activities in the prevention and management of health. IEC is a general acronym for the word Information Education and Communication. "The concept of IEC in health education and promotion is based on the premise that effective dissemination of information is crucial in the promotion of health in all dimensions. When carefully carried out, health communication strategies help to foster positive health practices individually and institutionally, and can contribute to sustainable change towards healthy behaviour" (WHO, 2001). In another vein, IEC has been described as a general term for communication activities to promote a variety of issues including health, sanitation and child rights. It is an approach based on the need to make all concerned to become more effective communicators. The promotion of effective IEC involves the identification of a mix of channels of communication such as the mass media, print media and traditional forms of entertainment (UNICEF, 2002). IEC is basically a process of working with individuals, communities and societies to develop communication strategies to promote positive behaviours, which are appropriate to their settings (UNESCO, Bangkok, 2005). Bertrand, Janet and Kincaid, Lawrence (1996) defines process of health awareness materials through grouped IEC activities under the following: Mass Media; Radio/TV, Newspaper/Magazine, Cinema/ Video, Boards/Posters, Pamphlets/Books Flip Charts and Folk Songs (Table 2.2).

Table 2.2: Health Awareness Activities in Rayagada

Sl. No.	*Activities undertaken by ASHA*	*IEC/BCC Material*
1.	Registration of pregnant mother	•
2.	Counselling on ANC, PNC, safe delivery	•
3.	Accompany pregnant mother to hospital	•
4.	Distribution of IFA, Oral pills, ORS	•
5.	Distribution of DOTS	•
6.	Inform AWW/ANM on birth and death	•
7.	Help AWW in supplementary nutrition feeding	•
8.	Motivate for construction of latrines	•
9.	Help ANM for Immunization	•
10.	Education to Adolescents	•
11.	Motivate the couple for family planning	•

Source: CDMO, Rayagada.

One of the key components of the National Health Mission is to provide every village in the country with a trained Female Community Health Activist Anganwadi Worker, Accredited Social Health Activist (ASHA) and Auxiliary Nurse Midwife (ANM). ASHA working at grassroots level will lead to a self-sustaining health model for the tribal's. The primary health care infrastructure provides the first level of contact between the population and health care providers and forms the common pathway for implementation of all the health and family welfare programmes. It provides integrated promotive, preventive, curative and rehabilitative services to the population close to their hearth and home. A majority of the health care needs of the tribal population are taken care of either by the trained health personnel at the primary health care level or by their own traditional indigenous health practitioners at village level.

Traditional health care practice among the Kandha tribal generally relate to ecology, forest and nature and has deep-rooted linkages with their own culture, beliefs, superstitions and religious faith. Traditional and indigenous system of medicine still persists among the tribal people. Their unique traditional system of health care which has passed down from generation to generation is still the prevalent system. These traditional practices carry huge importance in the region where modern health care facilities are either not available or difficult to access.

The health seeking behaviour of the tribal groups is supposed to be highly associated with their beliefs, custom and practices, since, majority of the population in these societies are illiterate, poor and lacking modern health facilities. Health, disease and awareness are a continuous process and are interlinked with the health seeking behaviour of the community. The conceptualization and measurement of health and quality of life are gaining increasing attention in the health services. The present chapter has elaborated the insights tribal health and awareness among them. It is precisely their understanding of health and disease, which makes traditional health care practices indispensable for them.

Discussion

Health is a vital social sector which needs Government intervention especially in public health arena. In the modern society, educational status has attained an important place in depicting one's socio-economic condition. Education is helpful in bringing awareness towards social set-up and a consciousness about the happenings in and around the society and the whole world in vast sense. Education brings change in the society in a vast sense and is helpful in attitude and behaviour of people in general. Good health has always been an important concern of the people. There is a proverb saying "Health is Wealth". Health of an individual and of the society, when considered as an indicator of social and economic development of the nation, needs to be seen in its entirety and not in independence of other aspects of life that contribute to the overall development. Education is the key element in bringing about the political, economic and social changes needed to bring Health to All. In India important reasons behind the failure of the "Health for All" programme in India people are modernized medical practices provided by the government usually do not match with the respective culture of the Indian population and the government ignored the traditional healing system, even though they have better access to the people. Besides, acceptance of the modern medical system requires a minimum level of awareness of the people in terms of health care facilities available in the government health centres. Public Health is the science and art of promoting health, preventive disease and prolonging life through the organized efforts of society (WHO). The Public Health Wing of Odisha deals with prevention of epidemic diseases in the district. Malaria, blindness, leprosy, tuberculosis are major public health problems of the district. Many National Health Programmes such as National Anti-Malaria Programme (NAMP), Enhanced Malaria Control Programme (EMCP), AIDS Control Programme, National Leprosy Eradication Programme (NLEP), District Blindness Control Scheme (DBCS) and National Vector Borne Disease Control Programme (NVBDCP) are being implemented in the district. One of the prime objectives of any health system is to provide quality health care to its citizens. This is primarily done by strengthening the service delivery mechanism and improving systems and processes. In spite of this, the quality of the State Health Care varies widely across geographic areas, populations, and levels of care. The Health Policy 1983 and 2002 has emphasized on improving the health status of the people by creating efficient and effective public provisioning of health care in the country. The Government of Odisha through numerous programmes in the health sector claims that it is providing adequate, qualitative, preventive and curative health care to the people of the State as well as to ensure health care services to all, particularly to the disadvantaged groups like Scheduled Tribes, Scheduled Castes and the Backward Classes. The root causes of poor health continue to be poverty, social deprivation, low levels of literacy and inefficient health systems and infrastructure for health care and control of diseases, particularly communicable diseases. Socio-cultural inequities and barriers, insufficient assertion and demand for health care, inadequate geographic spread of service outlets and poor quality health care reduce access to and effectiveness of public services. The primary health care infrastructure provides the first level of contact between the population and health care providers and forms the common pathway for implementation of all the health and family welfare programmes. It provides integrated promotive, preventive, curative and rehabilitative services to the population close to their hearth and home. A majority of tribal population prefer to be cured in the nearby health centre or by the own traditional indigenous health provider (medicine man) at the village level. The health seeking behaviour of a large fraction of the population of the district still hover around traditional healers like Jaani, Disari, Beju, but due to the awareness programme and availability of modern health facilities at hands reach the majority have turned towards modern medicine. With the intervention of different disease control programmes the incidence of chronic disease has reduced but still the diseases like diarrhoea, cholera, measles, malaria, TB still pose a threat in the district. Tribal health is an important aspect of development and progress of the people. Tribal communities in general and the primitive tribal groups in particular are highly disease prone, and do not have required access to basic health facilities. The perception about health, disease and health seeking behaviour are not the same across culture. It varies from culture to culture as an integral part of ecology and culture ways. Human culture as a part of their cognitive development has complex ideas regarding causes of sickness and way of cure. This is the base of empirical medical systems that provide means for prevention and cure. This knowledge of prevention and cure of sickness is passed on from generation to generation. Public health is the science and art of promoting health, preventing disease and prolonging life through the organized efforts of society (WHO). Public health is a social and political concept aimed at improving health, prolonging life and quality of life among whole populations through health promotion, disease prevention and other forms of health intervention (Table 2.3).

With objective of health systems strengthening, as visualized under National Health Mission (NHM), one key strategic intervention are upgradation of health service delivery facilities so as to provide sustainable quality care with accountability and people's participation in IEC/BCC health activities circulated to all States. Additionally, an Information Education Communication IEC/BCC package is being worked out in consultation with IEC Division to promote the health information. It was also found that, though there was some IEC material on Reproductive Health, Maternal Health, Child Health

Table 2.3: Health Programme Awareness in Rayagada

Sl. No.	*Health Programme Indicator*	*Yes (%)*	*No (%)*
1.	IMNCI	8.38%	91.61%
2.	JSSK	18.06%	81.93%
3.	RBSK	0.64%	99.35%
4.	RKSK	1.29%	98.35%
5.	108	41.67%	58.70%
6.	102	23.87%	76.12%

Source: Present fieldwork.

(RCH), Adolescent Health, RBSK, RKSK, 108 Ambulance services, 102 Ambulance services displayed, these were sporadic and had no thought out strategy behind them to influence clients or service providers. BCC was lacking both in terms of any coordinated effort and content of messages. The popularity of IEC/BCC initiatives and their impact on the health of Kandha tribal populations all parts of district. To improve tribal population's access to health care and raise the quality of service provided, the World Bank. Raising awareness of health issues is the first step towards improving health outcomes. However, while public health programmes have frequently conducted Information, Education and Communication (IEC) campaigns; such as stressing the importance of hand washing, regular checkups, institutional deliveries, immunization etc.

Table 2.4: Health Seeking Behaviour Awareness in Rayagada

Sl. No.	*Behaviour Indicator*	*Yes (%)*	*No (%)*
1.	Toilet use	14.19%	85.80%
2.	Soap use	20%	80%
3.	Mosquito Net use	28.38%	71.61%
4.	Hand washing	24.51%	75.48%

Source: Present fieldwork.

Health sector reform under the National Health Mission (NHM), aims at increasing functional, administrative and financial autonomy of various field units. Under NHM, upgradation of health service delivery facilities for better community participation and accountability is strategized as a vehicle of flexible funding by the government to help raise the quality of care, by making the health service delivery system more responsive to meet people's needs with equitable access. With the help of Department of Health Research (DHR) and Indian Council of Medical Research (ICMR), the government should enable an environment for collaborating major research institutes for preparing a plan of action and methods and generating knowledge based health information system to achieve healthcare for all in India. There is a need to carry out reforms in accordance with the WHO framework for strengthening health systems.

Table 2.5: Household-wise Health Practice in Rayagada

Sl. No.	*Health Practice Indicator*	*Yes (%)*	*No (%)*
1.	Modern Health	138 (89.03%)	17 (10.96%)
2.	Traditional Health	124 (80%)	31 (20%)
3.	Modern and Traditional Health	74 (47.74%)	81 (52.25%)

Source: Present fieldwork.

To improve the content and quality of health messages and targeted them at specific tribal groups through the means appropriate to each. As Kandha tribal population find it difficult to navigate through the complexities of medical facilities. In partnership with local NGOs, counsellors who are often from tribal communities themselves have been placed at district hospitals to guide patients, explain doctor's prescriptions, help patients take advantage of welfare schemes and counsel them on preventive and promotive health behaviours. There is significant scope to expand these initiatives to regions that continue to be underserved or require additional inputs for improving tribal health outcomes.

Conclusion

Health is a prerequisite for human development and is an essential component for the well-being of the mankind the culture of community determinants the health behaviour of the community in general and individual members in particular the tribes in India. The relationship between culture and the health status of the population is interlinked hence last decades. Therefore, an anthropologist's role would be to mediate between health planners and health system on one side, and people, communities on the other. It is expected to act as an advocate for communities, as well ensure that health programmes are acceptable to them.

It is essential that health service planning and delivery in rural and remote areas takes account of these social factors, and recognizes the role of other sectors, such as housing, education, infrastructure, transport and maintaining the health of those who live in these communities. Finally, generalized all the opinions and suggestions towards health and health programmes people are ready to accept modern health practice but all Governments. health programmes not reached there. So, our Government has planned out for that and starts work for them as per guideline. Government covering all the social issues towards the health problem in community area and awareness creating among Kandha people's access to all types of community-based health services and programmes including health promotion, health plans, priority setting, evaluation and community capacity building.

Acknowledgements

A part of this chapter has been presented at the National seminar on "Role of Anthropology in Public Health", at Habra, West Bengal held on March 18-19, 2017. The author acknowledges the support of Department of Anthropology, Utkal University, Odisha.

References

Balgir, R.S. (2004), Dimensions of rural tribal health, Nutritional status of Kondh tribe and tribal welfare in Orissa: A biotechnological approach, Proceedings of the UGC sponsored National Conference on Human Health and Nutrition, 12-13th December, 2004, Thane, Maharashtra, pp. 45-47.

Behera, Deepak Kumar (2014). *Contemporary Society: Tribal Studies: Health in the Context of Tribal Culture*, (Vol. 9), New Delhi: Concept Publishing Company (P) Ltd.

Census (2011). Government of India.

Chaudhary, S.N. (2012). *Tribal Health and Nutrition,* New Delhi: Rawat Publications.

Chaudhury, Sukanta K. (2004). *Tribal Identity: Continuity and Change among Kondhs of Odisha,* Jaipur and New Delhi: Rawat Publications.

District Statistical Hand Book, Rayagada, Census 2011, Government of India.

Hahn, A. and Inhorn, M. (eds.) (2010). *Anthropology and Public Health,* 2nd ed., Bridging Differences in Culture and Society, New York: Oxford University Press.

Mohindra, K.S., Mukherjee, S., Khan, S. and Thresia, C.U. (2012). "Towards the next generation of public health research in India: A call for a health equity lens", *Journal of Epidemiology and Community Health*, Vol. 66, pp. 839-842.

Mukherjee, Amitava (2004). *Participatory Learning and Action, Monitoring and Evaluation and Participatory Monitoring and Evaluation*, New Delhi: Concept Publishing Company.

Patnaik, Nihar Ranjan (1992). *History and Culture of Khond Tribes*, New Delhi: Commonwealth Publishers.

Phadke, A. (2003). "Right to health care—Towards an agenda", *Economic and Political Weekly*, 38(41): 4308-4309.

Sankar, D., and Kathuria, V. (2004). "Health system performance in rural India efficiency estimates across states", *Economic and Political Weekly*, 39(13): 1427-1433.

Tribhuwan, Robin, D. (2004). *Health of Primitive Tribes*, New Delhi: Discovery Publishing House.

World Health Organization, 1995. *Decentralization and Health Systems Change: A Framework for Analysis.* WHO document WHO/SHS/NHP/95.2. Geneva.

3

Challenges of Health Care and Sanitation among the Birhor of Hazaribag, Jharkhand

Divya Bharti and *Ganga Nath Jha*

Introduction

There are thirty two tribal groups in Jharkhand, among these eight are Particularly Vulnerable Tribal Groups (PVTGs) Birhor is one of the primitive and vulnerable tribal group in eight PVTGs of Jharkhand. Birhors are present mainly in the area of Hazaribag, Ramgarh, Gridih, Dhanbad, Bokaro, Gumla, Ranchi and Singhbhum districts in Jharkhand. According to Census 2011 total population of Birhors in Jharkhand is 10,726, in which 5,472 are male and 5254 are female. Total population of Birhor in Hazaribag district is 2049 in which 1039 are male and 1010 are female.

The Birhors affirm that they have descended from the Sun. The term Birhor in Mundari means a woodman or a chop cutter (lords of the jungles). The Birhors are largely a nomadic tribe with no fixed habitation; they roam about from forest to forest in search of subsistence. The Birhors are divided into two classes—Uthlus (the wanderers) and Janghis (the settlers). The Uthlu Birhors are always on the move, when the food supply in a particular area is exhausted, they move on to another jungle. But presently, it appears that in Jharkhand all Birhors are settled in government colonies or Tanda (village). Uthlu Birhors are not wanderers any more in Jharkhand; all Uthlus are settled. The Janghi Birhor on the other hand is of a more settled type. A few families, tired of wandering, have settled down on some hill top or on the outskirts of some forest. A few Janghi Birhors have cleared some land in the jungle for permanent cultivation, but the majorities are landless and live mainly by hunting and selling ropes. The Birhors move in small bands snaring monkeys, trapping hare, deer and other game or collecting rope fibres for making ropes for sale, also for collecting honey and bee-wax. The temporary Birhor settlements are known as *tanda*. These consist of at least half a dozen huts of conical shape, erected with leaves and branches. The household possessions traditionally consisted of earthen utensils, some digging implements, implements for hunting and trapping, rope making implements, baskets and so on. In recent times aluminium and steel have found their way into Birhor huts. After India's Independence in 1947, the government has attempted to settle the Birhors by giving them land, bullocks for cultivation, agricultural implements and seeds. Schools for children, rope making centre and honey collection training centres were started. Now, Birhor live settled life. But, still they depend on hunting, food gathering and minor food products, like bark of tree for rope-making, ethno-medicine, honey, leaf and fire wood. Birhors of Jharkhand are also known as rope-makers. Traditionally, they are making rope for neighbouring castes and tribes by the fibres of tree (*mohlan/chop chal*).

Objectives

The present study is a humble approach to explore the perception and practices of health behaviour and challenges along with socio-cultural profile of Birhor of Hazaribag.

Methodology

The research design of the present study incorporated the entire objective described above. The study used qualitative techniques to learn about the experiences, perception and practices of relevant health behaviour, the traditional healing practices of Birhor. The selection of villages for the study was made on the basis of availability of a Birhor tribal group. Key informant interview with auxiliary nurse midwife (ANM)/anganwadi worker (AWW)/traditional birth attendant (TBA), local registered medical practitioner (RMP), who practices in the village, traditional healers (village based) focus group discussion with eligible couples. Personal interviews were conducted upon randomly selected Birhor population. In this study both primary as well as secondary sources have been used. Research is mainly based upon response to a tailored questionnaire to collect data about their occupation and daily working schedule. Interview was taken to know traditional, cultural practice and change in culture. Observation, case study focus group discussions and photography have also been used. Secondary data was collected from library, archives etc. The schedule was filled in different areas, including health facilities, child health issues, maternal health, family health planning, immunization were main focus areas were studied by filling the schedule and observation. Total 46 household censuses were done from Kandsar and Sijua Birhor *tanda.*

Research Area

Two *tandas* are taken to an account—Kandsar Birhor tanda, and Sijua Birhor *tanda*. Kandsar Birhor *tanda* is situated in Katkamsandi Block and Sihua Birhor *tanda*, is in Ichak Block. Kandsar is situated 18 km south-west of Hazaribag on NH-100. Sijua is situated 12 km from Hazaribag headquarters on Hazaribag-Patna Road (NH-33). Thirty families reside in Kandsar and 16 families in Sijua (Tables 3.1 to 3.3).

Table 3.1: Birhor at a Glance

State	*Total Population*	*Male*	*Female*	*Total literacy*	*Male*	*Female*
Jharkhand	10,726	5,472	5,254	2,832	1,731	1,101

Source: Census 2011.

Table 3.2: District-wise Birhor Population

District	*Total Population*	*Male*	*Female*
Ranchi	791	421	370
Ramgarh	590	199	291
Hazaribag	2049	1039	1010
Chatra	2337	1204	1133
Giridih	554	273	281
Bokaro	305	171	134
Dhanbad	310	147	163
Deoghar	40	17	23
Koderma	1321	654	667
Khunti	56	25	31
Lohardagga	117	57	60
Latehar	192	105	87
Gumla	696	345	351
East Singhbhum	343	171	172

Source: Census 2011.

Table 3.3: Village Profile of Kandsar and Sijua Birhor Tandas

Name of village	*Total Households*	*Total Population*	*Male*	*Female*
Kandsar Birhor Tanda	30	83	41	42
Sijua Birhor Tanda	16	48	27	21

Source: Field Survey 2015-16.

Economic Status

Birhors depend on forests for their livelihood. They are hunters and food gatherers. For their economy they make *datun*, rope and for rope making material they depend on forests. They hunt hare, birds etc. They collect leaves and wood from forest. They also collect *Mahua* fruits in the season of *Mahua*. They dry the fruit for several purposes. They use *Mahua* as vegetable, medicines and also use for making drinks. They collect *Bhatua sag* and dry it. Everyday they use *bhatua sag* as their meal with rice. They use tree stems and leaves for making their traditional hut (*Kumba*). Their livelihood mainly depends on forest products, but today's scenario is little changed. They are living in transaction phase of occupation from food gathering and hunting to labour work. Birhors of Sijua Village are working as labour on crusher machine.

Table 3.4: Educational Institutions

Name of Village	*AWC*	*Primary School*
Kandsar Birhor Tanda	1	1
Sijua Birhor Tanda	1	1

Health Issues and Sanitation Problems

Nutritional status among Birhors of Hazaribag is very poor. They mostly take *Bhatua sag* and rice as their breakfast and lunch and sometimes *roti* in dinner. Majority of the tribal women are at risk of delivering low birth weight babies and have pregnancy complications. Some of the reasons for under-nutrition among tribal women could be poor diet intake, ignorance, early marriage, and high morbidity due to unhygienic practices and surroundings. Early marriage also causes health issues. Average age of marriage is reported 12 to 25 years and birth of first child 15 to 31. Under nutrition of mothers may be carried over to their children. Birhors are suffering from deficiency of Carbohydrate, Protein, Calcium, Vitamin and Iron. It

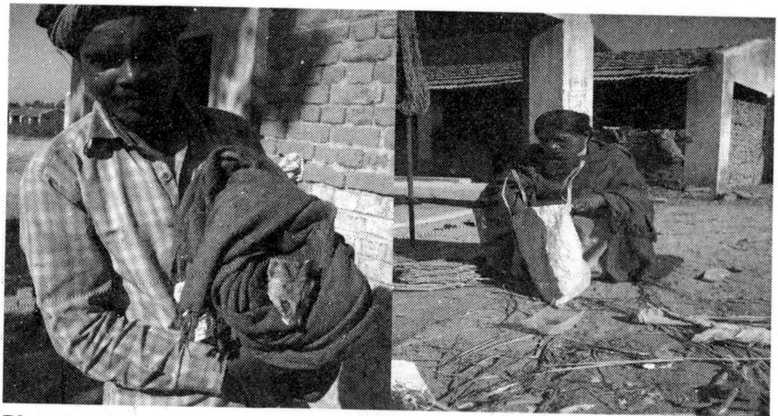

Plate 1: Birhor man going to sell kulhai (wild rabbit); Birhor woman preparing to go to local *haat* to sell *datun* (MFP).

affects on physical growth and health. Diseases like—Malaria, liver cirrhosis, are common among them. Water borne disease (Diarrhoea), skin disease like chicken pox and respiratory infection has been reported on 26 January, 2016 in Kandsar Birhor tanda. Children of age group 2 to 14 mostly suffer from chicken pox. Hence, there is a need to provide special attention to this group in improving their nutritional status by intervening appropriate health and nutrition programmes like nutrition education, iron supplementation, both during adolescence and during adulthood.

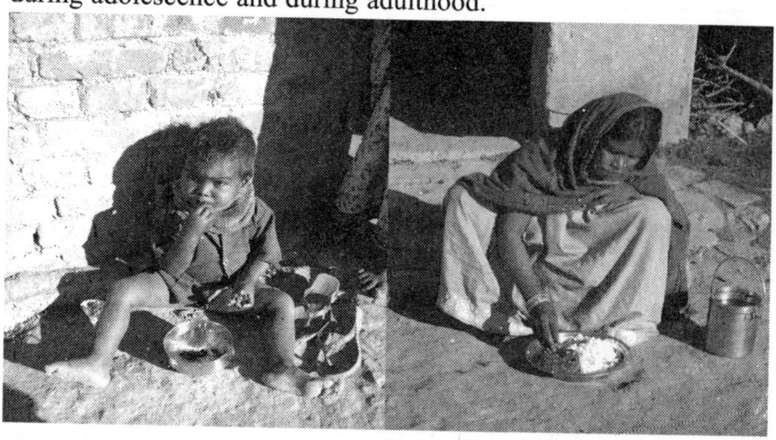

Plate 2: Birhor child and woman—taking food in unhygienic condition at Tauda (A *Birhor* village), Hazaribag.

Poor child rearing practices also cause health problems. Poor house and family management.

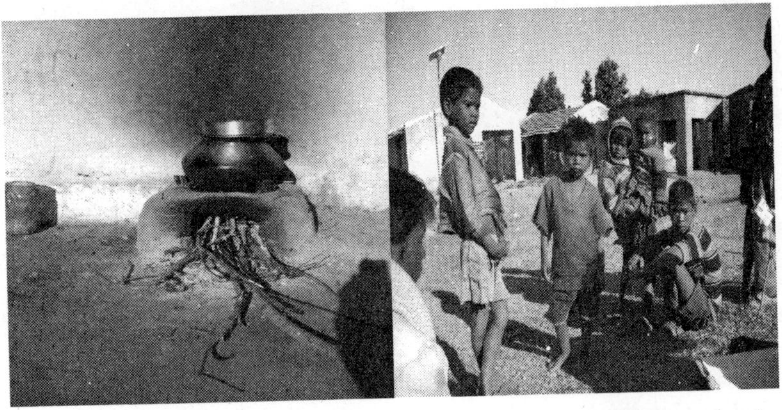

Plate 3: Preparation of food in traditional way; Birhor children playing in unhygienic ground.

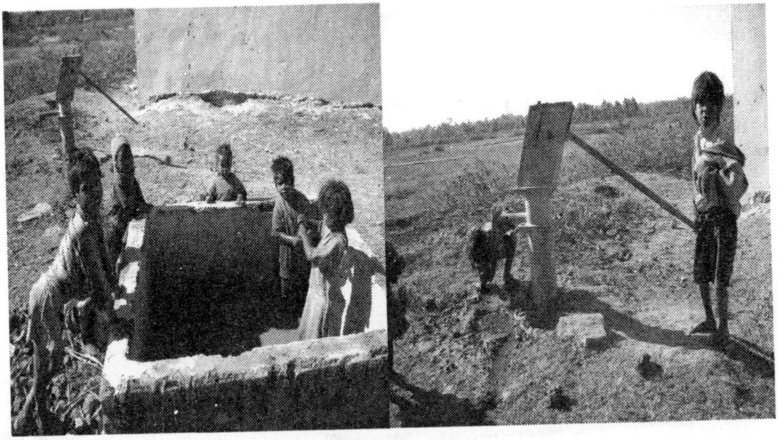

Plate 4: Birhor children playing in dirty and empty water tank; Lack of drainage system around hand pump.

Lack of habit of hygiene and sanitation are causes of health problems among them. They do not wash hand before taking food. They do not take bath because they have scarcity of cloths and they do not have money to buy soap. They do not use slipper or shoes.

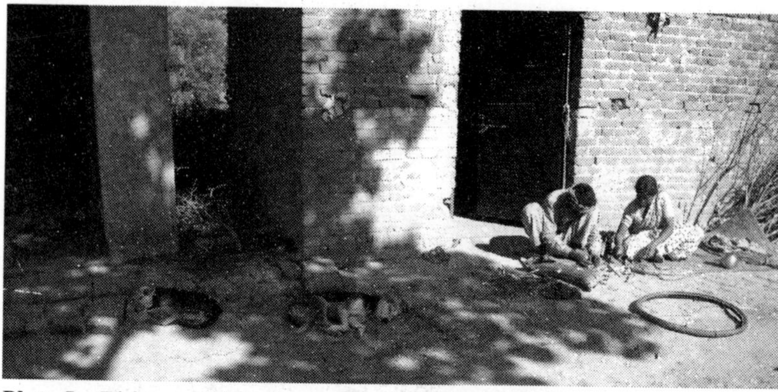

Plate 5: Birhor couple in front of Shabby Birsa/Indira Aawas.

They have only one room provided by the government according to Indira Gandhi Aawas Yojana. They do all their daily household work in a single room even they live with their pets in the same room.

Ignorance of Government Officials towards Birhors

Clean drinking water is not available in these villages. There are two hand-pumps in these villages one is in bad condition. They have Antyodaya Ration Card, but they do not get ration.

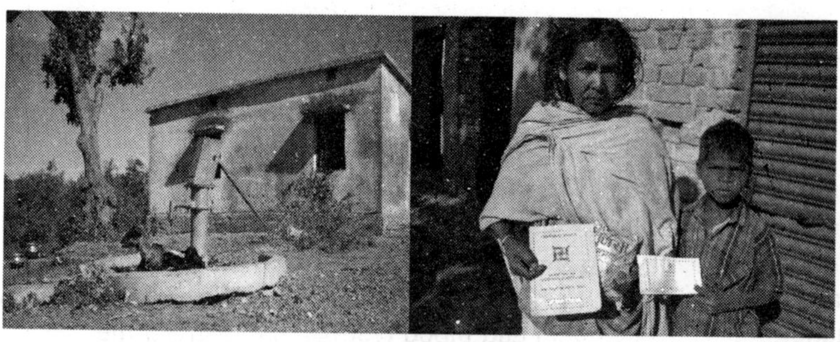

Plate 6: Dysfunctional hand pump in Kandsaar Tanda, Hazaribag, Jharkhand; Birhor woman and child with BPL and Antyodaya Card.

They are habituate of drinking *Hadiya*. They consume alcohol more than their meals. Whatever ration they get from Antyodaya Ration Card they sell it and drink alcohol.

Superstition and Practice of Ethno-medicine in Disease

They depend on medicine-man for treatment of all types of diseases and Ethno-medicine, but Ethno-medicine is not suitable for every type of diseases and Mal-nutrition.

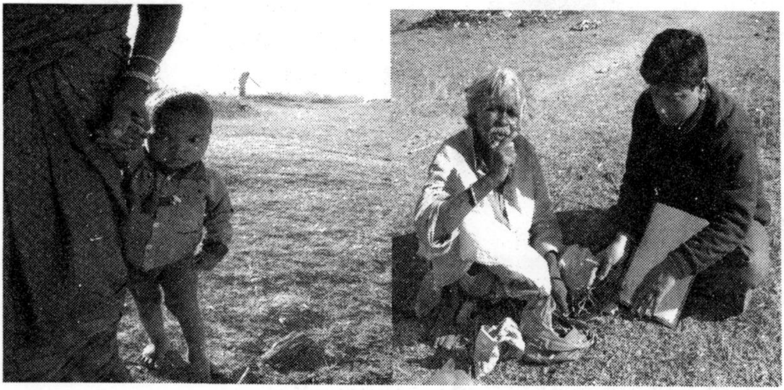

Plate 7: Author taking interview of Ethno-medicine expert of Birhor Community.

Case Study-1

Sunita Birhorin, age 24, of Kandsar Birhor Tanda went forest to collect forest product and deliver her child in the forest. She cut her child umbilical cord by sickle (*Hasua*) and after some time she came back.

Case Study-2

Sukri Birhorin, age 26 of Sijua Birhor Tanda said that in the colony the Birhor are strongly believe in traditional healer which can treat all diseases. They go to modern health providers for treatment only in critical cases. She said that when a woman has problems related to menstruation like abdomen pain and blood clotting she is given the juice of a leaf known as *Pather Kucchi* (Coleus). She is also given the juice of a flower called Jab. She said that the health awareness and level of knowledge among the Birhor people is very low. Miscarriages were also a common phenomenon in the colony.

The health problems of any community are influenced by interplay of various factors including social, economic and political one. The common beliefs, customs, practices related to health and disease in turn influence the health seeking behaviour of the community. There is a consensus agreement that the health status of the tribal population is very poor and worst among the primitive tribes, because of their isolation, remoteness and being largely unaffected by the development process going on in the country. The goal of any community or health care provider for that matter should be to prolong the number of years of healthy life of the population it represents or cares for. With that goal in mind people, social infrastructures, Government aid to those most in need and investigation of disease outbreaks may all play a role in the public's health. The causes of health inequalities lie in the social, economic, and political mechanisms that lead to social stratification according to income, education, occupation, gender and race or ethnicity. The above chapter indicating that the Birhor are still far away from the modern civilization and developments. In spite of the tremendous advancement in the field of preventive and curative medicine, the health care delivery services in the Birhor are still poor and need to be strengthened in order to achieve the goal of Health for All.

Conclusion and Suggestion

- Birhor are the man of jungle. They spend their livelihood from hunting and gathering forest products. But government has settled them in a small house of one room far from the nature in a colony without teaching them new occupational skill.
- Now-a-days, they are also working as labours and tractor drivers. Government should provide them skill training in a proper way.
- In jungle they use to wear very little cloth but in these colonies they have only single cloth to wear. So, they do not take bath regularly.
- When they were living in jungle they use to take rice beer which was made by them. But now, they came in contact with other people and they are addicted of alcohol.
- They are suffering from skin diseases, because they are not aware of sanitation.
- They depend on Ethno-medicine for all types of disease.
- Medical team should visit to these villages at least once a month.
- Government should make CCD plan with time to time monitoring and implement it in proper way.

- Drinking water should be provided to them.
- Government has provided them a room, but it is not in condition to live. All house need to be rebuild.
- They keep utensil in unhygienic place so, training should be given to make racks of mud, so that they can keep their utensils in hygienic place.
- Digital health card should be issued to them and time to time checkup should be done.

References

Balaji, L.N. (1995). *Health of Women, Children and Men in Tribal Areas—Focus for Consideration,* New Delhi: Concept Publishing Company, pp. 77-79.

Chaudhuri, B. (1992). "Health, religion and culture: The tribal situation", In: Chaudhari, Buddhadeb, *Tribal Transformation in India,* Vol. 2, New Delhi: Inter-India Publications, pp. 211-215.

Friis, R.H. and Seller, T.A. (1999). *Epidemiology for Public Health Practice.* 2nd edition. USA, Gaithersburg: M.D. Aspen Publication.

Health of Tribal Population in India: Results of Some ICMR Studies. (1988) Indian Council of Medical Research, New Delhi.

Mohanta, B.K. and Sinha, V.K. (2012). *Traditional Knowledge System and Technology in India.* Delhi: Pratibha Prakashan, pp. 55-80 and 189-196.

Park, J.E. and Park, J.K. (1983). "Healthcare of the community", In: K. Park *Text Book of Social Medicine*, Jabalpur: Banarsideas Bhanot, pp. 534-535.

Prasad, N. (1961). *The Land and People of Tribal Bihar.* Ranchi: Bihar Tribal Research Institute.

Regional Conference Proceedings at Djakarta Indonesia, Revitalizing Primary Health Care, (2008). Published by World Health Organization, Regional Office for South-East Asia, New Delhi.

Report on Scheduled Tribes, Scheduled Areas and Tribal Areas in India. (1998), Published by Ministry of Social Justice and Empowerment (Tribal Division), Government of India.

Roy, S.C., (1925). *The Birhor—A Little Known Jungle Tribe of Chhotanagpur, India*, Ranchi: The G.E.L. Mission Press, Printed by Elias Purti, Published by the Author Man in India, Church Road, Ranchi.

Sachchidanand (1965). *Peoples of Tribal Culture in Bihar.* Calcutta: Firma K.L. Mukhopadhyay.

Singh, K.S. (2008). *People of India, Bihar including Jharkhand,* Vol. XVI, Part 1. Kolkata: Anthropological Survey of India, pp. 460-462 and 641-644.

Vidyarthi, L.P. (1976). *Tribal Culture of India.* New Delhi: Concept Publishing Company.

Part-II

Epidemiology of Non-Communicable Diseases

4

Social Determinants of Cardiovascular Diseases

Arnab Ghosh

Introduction

The relationship between cardiovascular diseases (CVD) and risk factors such as high blood pressure, cholesterol, smoking, diabetes and physical inactivity has been the subject of extensive study, resulting in an abundance of literature. On the other hand, fewer studies have documented social determinants such as working conditions, housing, or social relationships. In this chapter, we suggest that social determinants should not only be juxtaposed with traditional risk factors acting directly on CVD, but also be examined as underlying determinants of some CVD, and, indeed, as factors acting along causal chains, influencing the incidence and management of traditional risk factors as well as the management of acute coronary events. The goal of this review is not to be exhaustive in discussing all social determinants of CVD, but to emphasise their variety as well as the mechanisms through which they act upon disease, in the light of recent works.

Why Social Determinants have Emerged and Why They Need to be Explored ?

The broad mechanisms involved in the development of CVD, including biological and behavioural risk factors, availability of treatments, and an overall fall in CVD rates in industrialised countries, are now well understood. Despite this, there are three issues that highlight the fact that it is essential we improve our knowledge of cardiovascular disease determinants: firstly, social inequalities in health have not disappeared over recent decades, in fact if anything they have increased; secondly, dramatic increases in CVD incidence have been observed after certain rapid social changes, such as in Eastern Europe in the nineties, after the fall of the Soviet Union; and finally, an increase in the incidence of CVD has been observed among some disadvantaged groups (Bourbonnais, Brisson, Malenfant and Vézina, 2005). In France, whereas in many countries of the world, social inequalities in mortality are higher among men than women, a change has been observed in terms of cardiovascular mortality, with higher inequalities emerging among women than among men. Changes in traditional risk factors do not explain this shift, which may actually be related to societal changes in the role of women at work (Bosma, Peter, Siegrist and Marmot, 1998).

Social Determinants of Health (SDH)

Social Determinants of Health (SDH) can be understood as the social conditions in which individuals live and work; conditions that are shaped by the distribution of power, income and resources, as much on a global and national level as on a local level. The study of these SDH is intended not only to demonstrate the impact of social context on health, but also the mechanisms *via* which these determinants act on health. This concept first arose in the seventies, when critics suggested that research and public policy should focus more on the societies within which individuals live than on the individuals themselves. It was a move away from a service provided to people when they were ill and towards a public health programme that would help them to stay healthy. SDH condition the physical, social, economic and personal resources an individual has available to them for meeting their needs and aspirations and adapting to their environment (Jood, Redfors, Rosengren, Blomstrand, C. and Jern, 2009).

A scientific debate separates those who believe that psychosocial mechanisms are keys, who accord importance to perceptions and social relationships, and those who insist on the importance of "objective", material conditions. The materialist hypothesis accords a predominant role to material conditions and their consequences on health. The approach concentrates on access to water, food, and chemical and physical exposure. Under this hypothesis, the "health behaviour" of an individual is considered more to be the product of social structures than a matter of individual responsibility. On the other hand, the psychosocial explanation postulates that material conditions have less influence on health than the psychological "stress" associated with the perception of a socio-economic disadvantage (in developed societies, at any rate) (Blakely and Woodward, 2000).

However, the two approaches, psychosocial and materialist, are not conflicting ones. In 2007, working conditions for employees and labourers in France were characterised by physically strenuous work and exposure to harmful physical and chemical factors, all of which are considered material factors (Jood, Redfors, Rosengren, Blomstrand and Jern, 2009). At the same time, studies on workplace organisation have demonstrated the importance of psychosocial explanations (e.g. such as the effort-reward imbalance model), which should not be considered as individual factors: we must understand how a workplace structure, which can be adjusted, translates into individual experience.

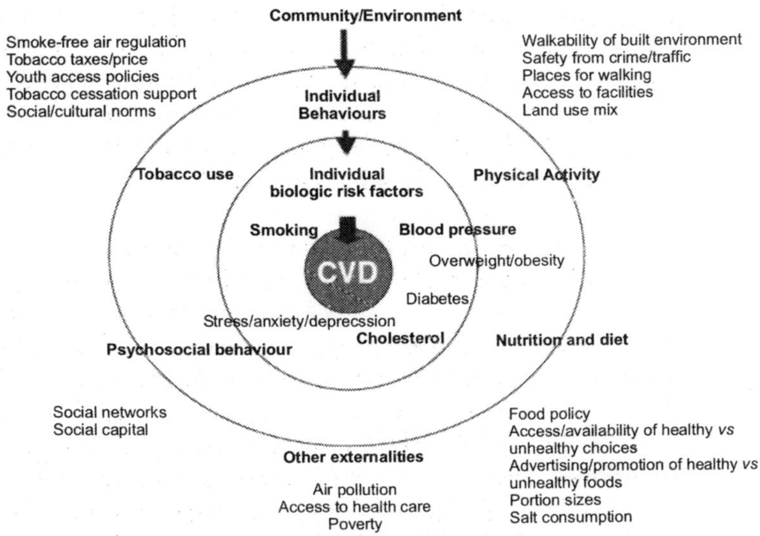

Fig. 4.1: Environmental factors that have been linked to human behaviours and established risk factors that cause cardiovascular disease

Social Determinants: What are the Key Factors?

The relationship between social determinants and CVD has been observed in many studies. We will focus on some main categories of social determinants of CVD: professional context (working conditions and access to a job), social relationships and isolation, geographic environment and "ethnicity". Social determinants have been shown to be related to various CVDs in various ways (Kreatsoulas and Anand, 2010). Indeed, from an epidemiological point of view, psychological stress has been linked to the development of cardiovascular risk factors such as hypertension and atherosclerosis. Self-perceived stress, as well as stress-related measures such as sense of coherence, has also been associated with stroke (Kreatsoulas and Anand, 2010).

Unemployment and Job Instability

The high mortality rate of the unemployed compared with those engaging in a professional activity is only partially explained by selection effects. An unstable situation, whether it involves unemployment or the fear of losing a job, has various effects on cardiovascular health (Lynch, Smith, Kaplan and House, 2000). These effects may also impact those in other types of unstable employment, such as fixed-term contracts, involuntary part-time work, seasonal work and internships. Restructuring operations have consequences not only on the individuals who find themselves unemployed, but also on the "survivors". Between 1993 and 2000, during a period of rapid growth in unemployment in Finland, cardiovascular mortality within companies in four towns increased by 50 per cent where staff reductions of eight to 18 per cent were made and by 100 per cent where the reduction was over 18 per cent, compared with companies where no staff cuts were made. Selection effects linked to health were excluded (Lynch, Smith, Kaplan and House, 2000).

Social Isolation

Social Isolation considerably increases the risk of death due to myocardial infarction. Increased overall and cardiovascular mortality rates have been observed where no social support network exists, more consistently in men than in women. These data on the effect of social relationships on overall and cardiovascular mortality rates have been confirmed by a recent meta-analysis. The association is more or less marked according to the social relationship measurement. The odds-ratio is higher for complex measurements of social integration than for binary measurements (living alone *versus* other arrangements). Multiple mechanisms are suggested, involving instrumental support (money and other help), emotional support, encouragement to access medical and preventative care, and a direct neurohormonal effect. Social networks, depending on the number of social contacts, friends, family members, work colleagues or neighbours an individual has and the social support that they can provide, have both a material and psychosocial impact, since their support may involve not only communication and emotional support, but also material or financial assistance (Marmot and Wilkinson, 2001).

Geographical Location

Links between CVD, mortality or hospitalisations, and short and long term fluctuation in atmospheric pollution relate not only to particulate matter, but also to ozone, carbon monoxide, nitrogen dioxide and sulphur dioxide. However, the distribution of populations with regard to pollution is not random. Due to property prices, populations of a low socio-economic status (SES) are more exposed to pollution (Marmot and Wilkinson, 2001). A Canadian cohort study confirms that exposure to environmental pollutants and traffic pollution explains, at least in part, the social gradient in health that has been observed. Cardiovascular risks, in particular an increased risk of myocardial infarction in the short-term associated with low temperatures, have been well-documented. Being able to heat the home, the quality of the insulation and therefore, the temperature inside the home seem to play a major role. A British study suggests that green spaces also have a beneficial effect. The inequality gradient was reduced by the presence of green spaces, even after stratification based on the area's level of deprivation.

Discrimination and Ethnicity

In France, questions of ethnicity in national statistics spark lively debate. It is worth defining ethnicity as a complex and changing social phenomenon that involves imposed categories as well as self-assigned identity. The majority of immigrants and their descendants belong to disadvantaged social categories. The issue is whether various types of discrimination, related to skin-colour, place of birth or surname, may have a detrimental effect on health beyond that of their social group (e.g., education and profession) and material quality of life (Saurel-Cubizolles, Chastang, Menvielle, Leclerc, Luce, 2009). Epidemiological indicators must specify the different types of discrimination encountered, and distinguish discrimination perceived individually *versus* that perceived by the group, and the fear of discrimination *versus* actual discrimination.

A United States review of published works shows a link between hypertension and institutional racism (Saurel-Cubizolles, Chastang, Menvielle, Leclerc, Luce, 2009). It would be helpful to undertake similar studies on discrimination in more European countries.

Interaction of Genetics, Biology and Social Environment

A 30-year study conducted on 144 nuns and 138 controls living around a monastery in Italy illustrates the societal effect and its interaction with the environment. For the nuns, almost their entire lives were spent in complete isolation and near-silence. Although urinary salt excretion in the two groups of individuals remained similar throughout the study, blood pressure in the control group increased with age, whilst that of the nuns remained constant. After 30 years, the difference in blood pressure was 30/15 mmHg. The effect of a high salt intake is, therefore, reduced by a life in this distinctive environment, which features lack of stress, silence and isolation from society (Surtees, Wainwright, Luben, Wareham, Bingham, and Khaw, 2007). There are concrete arguments to suppose that the social environment alters gene expression, however, this approach does not resolve the great problem of social epidemiology, that of characterising social environment.

Conclusion

There are many social determinants of CVD. They are found largely outside the healthcare and preventative healthcare systems; but, it is important to think in terms of chains of cause and effect, which enable us to see these determinants at work within the system of curative and preventative care, including in the management of traditional risk factors.

References

Blakely, A.B. and Woodward, A.J. (2000). "Ecological effects in multi-level studies", *J. Epidemiol Community Health.* 54: 367-74.

Bosma, H., Peter, R., Siegrist, J. and Marmot, M. (1998). "Two alternative job stress models and the risk of coronary heart disease". *Am. J. Public Health.* 88: 68-74.

Bourbonnais, R., Brisson, C., Malenfant, R. and Vézina, M. (2005). "Health care restructuring, work environment, and health of nurses". *Am. J. Ind. Med.*, 47: 54-64.

Jood, K., Redfors, P., Rosengren, A., Blomstrand, C. and Jern, C. (2009). "Self-perceived psychological stress and ischemic stroke: A case-control study". *BMC Med.*, 7:8.

Kreatsoulas, C., and Anand S.S. (2010). "The impact of social determinants on cardiovascular disease". *Can. J. Cardiol.,* 26:8C-13C.

Lynch, J.W., Smith, G.D., Kaplan, G.A. and House, J.S. (2000). "Income inequality and mortality: Importance to health of individual income, psychosocial environment, or material conditions". *BMJ.*, 320:1200-4.

Marmot, M. and Wilkinson, R.G. (2001). "Psychosocial and material pathways in the relation between income and health: A response to Lynch", *et al.*, *BMJ.,* 322:1233-6.

Saurel-Cubizolles, M.J., Chastang, J.F., Menvielle, G., Leclerc, A. Luce, D., EDISC group (2009). "Social inequalities in mortality by cause among men and women in France". *J. Epidemiol. Community Health,* 63:197-202.

Surtees, P.G., Wainwright, N.W.J., Luben, R.L., Wareham, N.J., Bingham, S.A. and Khaw, K.T. (2007). "Adaptation to social adversity is associated with stroke incidence-evidence from the EPIC-Norfolk prospective cohort study." *Stroke.* 38:1447-53.

5

Effect of Metabolic Risk Factors and Family History on Diabetes in Asian Indian Population

Riddhi Goswami, Indrani Lodh, and *Mithun Das*

Introduction

The prevalence of diabetes is rapidly increasing all over the world at an alarming rate. The major driver of the epidemic is the more common form of diabetes, namely type 2 diabetes mellitus (T2DM), which accounts for more than 90 per cent of all diabetes cases. India is the worst hit country with an estimated 32 million people with diabetes in the year 2000 and this number is steadily increasing and set to reach about 70 million by the year 2025. Asian Indians are ethnically predisposed to diabetes and tend to develop the disease much earlier and have a pre-inflammatory state that may contribute to their increased risk (Mohan *et al.*, 2007; Huizinga and Rothman, 2006; Wild *et al.*, 2004).

Metabolic risk factors such as dyslipidemia, hypertension, abdominal obesity and impaired blood glucose regulation when coupled with family history and genetic predisposition can provide important insights into the prevalence of T2DM and their inheritance to the next generation. Family history of diabetes (FHD) is not only a risk factor for the disease, but is also important for relevant awareness programmes to ensure risk-reducing behaviours for target population. It may be used as a screening tool for detection and/or prevention of diabetes (Hariri *et al.*, 2006). In a study among the adult Chinese, it was observed that sufficient physical activity and negative FHD might jointly reduce the risk of developing T2DM

(Xu *et al.*, 2012). In the US population, FHD showed significant, independent, and graded association with the prevalence of T2DM. This association opens up the possibility of formally adding family history to public health strategies aimed at detecting and preventing the disease (Valdez *et al.*, 2007; Das *et al.*, 2012).

Insulin Receptor Substrate (IRS) molecules are key mediators in insulin signalling and play a central role in maintaining basic cellular functions such as growth, survival and metabolism. Polymorphisms in the IRS gene family are associated with insulin resistance. Of four genes in the IRS system (IRS1, IRS2, IRS3, and IRS4), IRS1 and IRS2 play important roles in glucose metabolism (Malik *et al.*, 2005). C-reactive protein (CRP) is widely known to be a sensitive circulating marker of inflammation and is associated with increased risk of CVD. Inflammation is also associated with insulin resistance and hence the development of diabetes (Sesti *et al.*, 2001; Dehghan *et al.*, 2007).

Pregnancy is characterized by peripheral insulin resistance and gestation diabetes mellitus develops if insulin secretion fails to overcome insulin resistance. It is assumed that intrauterine exposure to an excess of glucose causes permanent foetal changes. Although maternal glucose freely crosses the placenta, maternal insulin does not. In pregnancies complicated by diabetes, this would lead to greater birth weight and increased risk of development of T2DM in later life (Dabela, 2007; Tam *et al.*, 2014; Ayaz *et al.*, 2014).

Asian Indians are ethnically predisposed to diabetes and tend to develop the disease much earlier and have a pre-inflammatory state that may contribute to their increased risk. These factors when coupled with family history and genetic predisposition can shed important insights into the prevalence of type 2 diabetes and their inheritance to the next generation. The objective of our study includes determination of the prevalence of metabolic risk factors and genetic polymorphisms among the obstetric Asian Indian population, with respect to their family history. In this study, we have selected two candidate genes for studying their polymorphism status—IRS-1 (Insulin receptor substrate-1) and IRS-2 (Insulin receptor substrate-2).

The main objective of the study was to assess the role of family history as a risk factor in the prevalence of T2DM and their inheritance to the next generation with respect to biochemical and genetic factors in Asian Indian population by a longitudinal study throughout the gestation period.

Materials and Methods

Study Population: This is a longitudinal follow-up study and present study was being done in continuation with the earlier work. The medical history of the patient's family was recorded. Determination of presence or absence of other risk factors—high cholesterol levels, cigarette smoking, hypertension, diabetes in first-degree relatives (biological parents, siblings, and offspring) was recorded. The present study was conducted on 180 healthy (non-diabetic, normotensive) adult Asian Indian women [including 100 with and 80 without family history of diabetes (FHD)] living in and around Kolkata, India. This sample size was sufficient to test all the research hypotheses at the 5 per cent level of significance. During the gestation period they were studied twice, first within 12 weeks and second by 30 weeks. They were then followed up till delivery. During delivery both mothers' venous blood and cord blood were collected to estimate the metabolic variables and genetic polymorphisms of the respective mothers and their new born babies. Institutional Ethics Committee of Heritage Institute of Technology had approved the study and written consent was taken prior to the actual commencement of the study.

Anthropometric Measurements: Demographic profiles including name and date of birth were obtained from participants. Subjects' age to the nearest month was ascertained subsequently from date of birth. Informed consent was obtained from participants prior to the actual commencement of the study. Height was measured to nearest 0.1 cm with a Martin's Anthropometer and weight to the nearest 0.5 kg with a portable weighing machine in light clothing and bare feet.

Blood Pressure Measurements: Left arm systolic (SBP) and diastolic (DBP) blood pressure was taken from each participant with the help of an Omron M1 digital electronic blood pressure/pulse monitor (Omron Corporation, Tokyo, Japan). Two blood pressure measurements were taken and averaged for analysis. A third measurement was taken when the difference between the two measurements was ≥ 5 mmHg, and a subsequent mean was calculated. A five minute relaxation period between measurements was

Cholesterol, VLDL-Cholesterol, Fasting Blood Glucose and Blood Pressure, both at the gestational period of 12 weeks and 30 weeks. It indicates that family history plays an influencing metabolic factors and triggering the risk factors early in the gestational phase leading to complications in adult life.

Comparison of subjects in the CRP levels between the same groups also revealed a statistically significant difference in subjects with a positive FHD and high CRP levels in comparison to normal cases (Table 5.2).

Table 5.2: Difference in C-reactive Protein (CRP) by FHD

Family History of T2DM	*C-Reactive Protein*			
	Normal (< 0.6 mg/dl)	*High (>0.6 mg/dl)*	*Total*	
Both/Either	36	64	100	*p = 0.0109*
None	38	42	80	
Total	**74**	**106**	**180**	

Source: Author's Study.

Comparison of birth outcomes in terms of birth weights was done between subjects with and without a positive family history of T2DM and high CRP levels (Table 5.3), which revealed a significant difference between the two groups. This shows that family history and perturbations in the gestational period are reflected in the birth outcomes, affecting the next generation (Table 5.4). It is evident from

Table 5.3: Differences in Birth Outcomes (Birth Weight in kg) by FHD and CRP of the Mothers

Mothers' status	*Birth Weight (Kg)*				*ANOVA*
	Under weight (< 2.5 kg)	Normal (2.5-4.2 kg)	Overweight (>4.2 kg)	Total	
Positive Family History with High CRP	25	17	21	63	p = 0.0252
No Family history with Normal CRP	17	22	10	49	
Total	**42**	**39**	**31**	**112**	

Source: Author's Study.

Table 5.4: Differences in C-Reactive Protein (CRP) of the Babies by Mothers' CRP and FHD

CRP of the Babies	*Mothers with +FHD and high CRP (n = 63)*	*Mothers with FHD and normal CRP (n = 49)*	*ANOVA*
Mean	0.47	0.26	P < 0.001
SD	± 0.088	± 0.021	

Source: Author's Study.

the results that there is a significant difference in inflammatory status in those newborns whose mothers have a positive FHD compared to their normal counterparts.

The IRS-1 and IRS-2 genotypes were assessed on the basis of their prevalence among high CRP and FHD (Table 5.5). It was seen that there is no significant association of IRS-1 polymorphisms with FHD and CRP status, although, the presence of GA allele is much higher than GG and AA. The same observation holds true for IRS-2, but there is a strong association between the DD allele with FHD and CRP status, which proves its future potential as a biomarker.

Table 5.5: I/D Genotype Show a Close Association with Subjects with Positive Family History of MS and High CRP Values

Mother's Status	*Subjects with IRS-1 genotypes*			*Subjects with IRS-2 genotypes*		
	GG	*GA*	*AA*	*GG*	*GD*	*DD*
+FHD and high CRP (n = 63)	24	29	10	12	4	37
–FHD and low CRP (n = 49)	23	26	0	13	10	26

Source: Author's Study.

Discussion

Evidence suggests that FHD by itself is most useful for predicting T2DM when the disease is premature, that is, it occurs at younger ages than would be expected. It has been mentioned that FHD information in combination with other known risk factors could be used to provide more personalized information about our risk for such diseases (Yoon *et al.*, 2002). Yang *et al.*, 2010, further suggested that adding FHD could provide significant improvements in detecting undiagnosed diabetes; however, it needs further validation with larger cross-sections of population. In another study (Valdez *et al.*, 2007), it was found that not only the adults, but even the young population with a positive FHD showed signs of increased risk for these conditions which indicates the importance of family history approach to screening for children at risk of T2DM and CVD.

In the present study, it was found that individuals with positive family history of diabetes had significantly higher prevalence of metabolic risk factors and its confounding factors as compared to their counterparts during pregnancy, which is also affecting their next generation leading to childhood obesity. It can be stated that +FHD and CRP status plays an important role in triggering the activation of metabolic risk factors during the pregnancy period, and this could be one of the major factors for development of T2DM and metabolic syndrome in the next generations. These findings suggest that family history could be used as a tool for genomic studies among the Asian Indians.

Although many different genes have been projected as diabetogenes, the present study focused on the IRS-1 and IRS-2 genes. The Gly972Arg polymorphism did not change the expression level of IRS-1 or the degree of insulin stimulated tyrosine phosphorylation of IRS-1, but the Arg 972 polymorphism interfere with the interaction between IRS-1 and PI3-kinase, possibly by altering the tertiary structure of IRS-1. For this explanation, the Arg 972 IRS-1 polymorphism may be responsible in the development of insulin resistance and diabetes by impairing the ability of insulin to activate the IRS-1/PI3-kinase/Akt signalling pathway, consequently leading to defects in glucose transport, glucose transporters translocation and glycogen synthesis (Ghufran and Hussain, 2015). We have not found any prominent association between IRS-1 polymorphisms and FHD or CRP, which is partially agreeable with earlier reports (Almind *et al.*, 1996; Hasniza *et al.*, 2014; Kovacs *et al.*, 2003; Kumar and Sharan, 2012; Porzio *et al.*, 1999).

We have seen a strong association of the IRS-2 D allele in subjects with positive FHD and high CRP status, which is in agreement with earlier studies. The exact molecular mechanism by which the non-conservative G1057D variant affects insulin action is not clear. However, it is hypothesized that this introduces a charged amino acid (D) in place of a neutral one (G) in the domain of IRS-2 molecule located in between two putative tyrosine phosphorylation sites (at positions 1042 and 1072) of the protein (Ayaz *et al.*, 2014; Mammarella *et al.*, 2000; Bodhini *et al.*, 2007). Therefore, alterations in downstream signalling through IRS-2 seem to be involved. In case of gestational diabetes mellitus (GDM), it remains to be determined which GDM-related factors interfere with IRS-2 signalling to make any functional significance of the polymorphism become apparent.

We know that the genetic polymorphisms and their association to the disease phenotype are ethno-specific in their expression; that is why it is important to interpret these results in conjunction with other parameters, as we have done in this case. It is evident from our study that individuals with a positive family history of diabetes and IRS-2 D allele have significantly higher risk of becoming affected by metabolic syndrome than their counterparts. It also suggests that family history could be used as an important tool for genomic studies on Asian Indian population. But, it is noteworthy that in developing countries like India, one should be cautious about the accuracy of self-reported family history data.

For majority of chronic diseases affecting public health such as CVD, T2DM, hereditary factors and hence family history is a major risk factor for these diseases. A major cause of these diseases is due to such factors as genetic susceptibility, shared environment and common behaviours (Yoon *et al.*, 2012). Even in clinically recognized medicine, family history has been diagnosed as a potent yet non-modifiable factor that may influence the probability of occurrence of such diseases. Even though family history has been recognized as a potent interpreter of such diseases, it has been seldom used in preventative medicine care so as to diagnose, detect and to develop preventive strategies (Scheuner *et al.*, 1997; Williams *et al.*, 2001). However, family history has been included in professional guidelines to assess health risk, initiate interventions and also influence behavioural changes. Genomic tools might provide further insights into such diseases, but the advantages of family history as a low cost tool which reflects shared genetic and environmental factors seems to have greater acceptability than those of other genomic tools. Even with such advantages, it seems the use of family history in public health has been poorly explored (Valdez *et al.*, 2010).

It has been observed in a study carried on adult Chinese population that sufficient physical activity and the absence of family history of diabetes might jointly negate the risk of developing hyperglycemia and T2DM (Xu *et al.*, 2012). Also, family history of diabetes in US population showed an indirect relationship between family history and prevalence of diabetes. This association not only highlights the importance of genetics and environmental predisposition in diabetes but also adds another dimension of adding family history to public health strategies aimed at detection and prevention of the disease (Valdez *et al.*, 2007). The family history of diabetes is a risk factor for the disease, but at the same time it provides valuable insights into risk awareness and risk-reducing behaviours. Hence, it may be used as a useful screening tool for detection and prevention of diabetes (Hariri *et al.*, 2006).

The major limitation of this polymorphism study was that it was performed on a relatively small sample size and, therefore, is not representative of the Asian Indian population. Large-scale, nationally representative data, which is actually lacking in India, would have provided a better insight into the role of IRS polymorphisms on the prevalence of T2DM coupled with FHD.

Conclusion

In conclusion, having observed that family history of diabetes (FHD) is indeed an important and independent risk factor for genomic studies of complex diseases like T2DM, efforts should be made towards translating this knowledge for use in public health programmes designed to detect and prevent diabetes. Once this is achieved, FHD should be incorporated into the screening and prevention programmes for T2DM as rigorously as possible to make these programmes significant and cost-effective.

Our study also suggests that patients carrying IRS-2 D allele may be a determinant in susceptibility to GDM. The etiology of gestational diabetes seems to involve a complex interplay of multiple genetic, environmental and immunologic factors. Although no single theory can explain all cases, from this preliminary study it seems that IRS-2 gene polymorphism may be associated with increased risk of GDM. However, the assessment of whether these alleles have a direct effect on disease susceptibility is not known. Further studies with larger sample size are needed to support our findings and to define more exactly the place of IRS-2 as a direct marker of the degree in glucose intolerance.

Acknowledgements

The authors wish to thank the authorities of Heritage Institute of Technology, Kolkata, for providing the infrastructural help and support. The authors are also indebted to all the participants who participated in the study.

References

Almind, K., Inoue, G., Pedersen, O., and Kahn, C.R. (1996). "A common amino acid polymorphism in insulin receptor substrate-1 causes impaired insulin signalling: Evidence from transfection studies", *J. Clin. Invest.*, 97(11): 2569 2575.

Ayaz, L., Celik, S.K. and Cayan, F. (2014). "The G1057D polymorphism of insulin receptor substrate-2 associated with gestational diabetes mellitus", *Gynecol. Endocrinol.*, 30(2):165-168.

Bodhini, D., Radha, V., Deepa, R., Ghosh, S., Majumdar, P.P., Rao, M.R.S. and Mohan, V. (2007). "The G1057D polymorphism of IRS-2 gene and its relationship with obesity in conferring susceptibility to type 2 diabetes in Asian Indians", *International Journal of Obesity,* 31:97-102.

Celik, S.K., Ates, N.A., Kucuk, M.U., Yalin, S. and Akbay, E. (2014). "The G1057D polymorphism of insulin receptor substrate-2 (IRS-2) gene with type 2 diabetes in the Turkish population", *The New Journal of Medicine,* 31: 168 171.

Dabelea, D. (2007). "The predisposition to obesity and diabetes in offspring of diabetic mothers", *Diabetes Care,* 30: S169-S174.

Das, M., Pal, S., and Ghosh, A. (2012). "Family history of type 2 diabetes and prevalence of metabolic syndrome in adult Asian Indians". *J. Cardiovasc Dis. Res.,* 3:104-108.

Dehghan, A., Hoek, M.V., Sijbrands, E.J.G., Stijnen, T., Hofman, A. and Witteman, J.C.M., (2007). "Risk of type 2 diabetes attributable to C-reactive protein and other risk factors", *Diabetes Care,* 30:2695-2699.

Ghufran, M.H. Asal and Hussain, M.K. (2015). "Association of insulin receptor substrate-1 gene polymorphism with insulin resistance in type 2 diabetes mellitus in Iraqi population", *Journal of Biology, Agriculture and Healthcare,* 5(2): 58-61.

Hariri, S., Yoon, P.W., Qureshi, N., Valdez, R., Scheuner, M.T. and Khoury, M.J. (2006). "Family history of type 2 diabetes: A population-based screening tool for prevention?" *Genet Med.*, 8:102-8.

Hasniza, Z.H., Mohd, M.B., Rosnani, H., Norlaila, M. and Wan, Z.W.N. (2014). "A prospective cohort study on IRS gene polymorphisms in type 2 diabetes mellitus patients during severe/acute hyperglycemia phase 1: Association with insulin resistance", *Trop J. Pharm. Res.*, 13(6):895-901.

Huizinga, M.M. and Rothman, R.L. (2006). "Addressing the diabetes pandemic: A comprehensive approach". *Indian J. Med. Res.*, 124(5):481-484.

Kovacs, P., Hanson, R.L., Lee, Y.H., Yang, X., Kobes, S., Permana, P.A., Bogardus C. and Baier, L.J. (2003). "The role of insulin receptor substrate-1 gene (IRS1) in type 2 diabetes in Pima Indians". *Diabetes,* 52(12):3005-9.

Kumar, R. and Sharan, N. (2012). "Analysis of codon 972 (gly → arg) polymorphism in IRS-1 gene in type 2 diabetic population", *J. Med. Biochem.,* 31: 234-238.

Malik, S., Wong, N.D., Franklin, S., Jose, P., Fairchild, C. and Chen, R. (2005). "Cardiovascular disease in U.S. patients with metabolic syndrome, diabetes, and elevated C-reactive protein", *Diabetes Care,* 28:690-693.

Mammarella, S., Romano, F., DiValerio, A., Creati, B., Esposito, D.L., Palmirotta, R., Capani F., Vitullo, P., Volpe, G., Battista, P., Loggia, F.D., Mariani-Costantini R., Cama, A. (2000). Interaction between the G1057D variant of IRS-2 and overweight in the pathogenesis of type 2 diabetes. *Human Mol. Gen.,* 9(17):2517-2521.

Mohan, V., Sandeep, S., Deepa, R., Shah, B., Varghese, C. (2007). "Epidemiology of type 2 diabetes: Indian scenario", *Indian J. Med. Res.,* 125(3): 217-230.

National Cholesterol Education Programme (NCEP) 2001. Expert Panel on Detection, Evaluation and Treatment of High Blood Cholesterol in Adults (Adult Treatment Panel III) Executive Summary of the third report. *JAMA,* 285:2486-97.

Porzio, O., Federici, M., Hribal, M.L., Lauro, D., Accili, D., Lauro, R., Borboni, P. and Sesti, G. (1999). The Gly972→Arg amino acid polymorphism in IRS-1 impairs insulin secretion in pancreatic beta cells. *J. Clin. Invest.,* 104(3):357 64.

Sesti, G., Federici, M., Hribal, M.L., Lauro, D., Sbraccia, P. and Lauro, R. (2001). "Defects of the insulin receptor substrate (IRS) system in human metabolic disorders", *FASEB J.*, 15(12):2099-111.

Scheuner, M.T., Wang, S.J., Raffel, L.J., Larabell, S.K., Rotter, J.I. (1997). "Family History: A comprehensive genetic risk assessment method for the chronic conditions of adulthood", *Am. J. Med. Genet.,* 71:315-24.

Tam, C.H.T., Wang, Y., Luan, J., Lee, H.M., Luk, AOY, Tutino, G.E., Tong, PCY, Kong APS, So, WY, Chan, JCN, Ma RCW. (2014). "Maternal history of diabetes is associated with increased cardiometabolic risk in Chinese", *Nutrition and Diabetes,* 4:1-11.

Valdez, R., Greenlund, K.J., Khoury, M.J. and Yoon, P.W. (2007). "Is family history a useful tool for detecting children at risk for diabetes and cardiovascular diseases. A public health perspective?" *Pediatrics,* 120 (Suppl 2): S78-86.

Valdez, R., Yoon, P.W., Liu, T., Khoury, M.J. (2007). "Family history and prevalence of diabetes in the U.S. population: The 6-year results from the

National Health and Nutrition Examination Survey (1999-2004)", *Diabetes Care,* 30:2517 22.

Valdez, R., Yoon, P.W., Qureshi, N., Green, R.F., Khoury, M.J. (2010). "Family history in public health practice: A genomic tool for disease prevention and health promotion", *Annu. Rev. Public Health,* 31:69-87.

Wild, S., Roglic, G., Green, A., Sicree, R. and King, H. (2004). "Global prevalence of diabetes: estimates for the year 2000 and projections for 2030", *Diabetes Care,* 27(5):1047-1053.

Williams, R.R., Hunt, S.X., Heiss, G., Province, M.A., Bensen, J.T. and Higgins, M., *et al.* (2001). "Usefulness of cardiovascular family history data for population-based preventive medicine and medical research (the Health Family Tree Study and the NHLBI Family Health Study)", *Am. J. Cardiol.,* 87:129 35.

Xu, F., Wang, Y., Ware, R.S., Tse, L.A., Dunstan, D.W., Liang, Y., Wang, Z., Hong, X. and Owen, N. (2012). "Physical activity, family history of diabetes and risk of developing hyperglycaemia and diabetes among adults in Mainland China", *Diabet Med.,* 29(5):593-99.

Yang, Q., Liu, T., Valdez, R., Moonesinghe, R., Khoury, M.J. (2010). "Improvements in ability to detect undiagnosed diabetes by using information on family history among adults in the United States", *Am. J. Epidemiol.,* 171:1079-89.

Yoon, P.W., Scheuner, M.T., Peterson-Oehlke, K.L., Gwinn, M., Faucett, A. and Khoury, M.J. (2002). "Can family history be used as a tool for public health and preventive medicine", *Genet. Med.,* 4:304-10.

6

An Epidemiology of Hypothyroidism in North East Indian Population

A Review

Kh Dimkhohoi Baite and *S. Yaiphaba Meitei*

Introduction

Thyroid Gland is one of the largest endocrine gland in the body located in the neck just below the prominence of thyroid cartilage, sometimes called Adams Apple. It is about two inches long and consists of two lobes—the right lobes and the left lobe, each about the size of half a plum. The thyroid is part of the endocrine system, which is made up of glands that produce, store, and release hormones into the blood stream so that the blood can reach the body's cell. The thyroid gland synthesizes and secretes two active hormones—thyroxine (T4) and tri-iodothyronine (T3). The function of the thyroid gland is regulated by Thyroid Stimulating Hormone (TSH) secreted by the anterior pituitary gland through stimulation by thyrotropin releasing hormone (TRH) secreted from Hypothalamus.

Thyroid diseases are, arguably, among the commonest endocrine disorders worldwide. It may come about through a number of different mechanisms. Among the various types of thyroid hormones dysfunction the most common form are hyperthyroidism and hypothyroidism. Autoimmune factors may cause either hyperthyroidism or hypothyroidism. The thyroid may also be affected by malignancies and congenital conditions. Thyroid Hormones dysfunction has been proved to be one of the emerging health concerns all over the world especially in high altitude places. Iodine deficiency may cause Hypothyroidism and Cretinism in childhood and goitre in adulthood. One of the most common thyroid disorders in women is hypothyroidism, which leads to clinical manifestations such as delay in sexual maturation and onset of puberty, reduced fertility, impaired mental function, heart disorders, reduced appetite, anaemia, constipation, decreased renal blood flow etc. Hypothyroidism is also a common endocrine disorder resulting from deficiency of thyroid hormone or, more rarely, from their impaired activity at tissue level. In hypothyroidism, the thyroid gland produce less amount of thyroid hormone, such subject eventually will lead to have lower metabolic rate and clinical manifestation such as overweight, fatigue, hypotension and depression.

Epidemiology of Hypothyroidism

Hypothyroidism is relatively a common disorder. The prevalence of hypothyroidism increases with age and is nearly 10 times more common in females than in males. A study conducted by American Thyroid Association states that about 20 million Americans have some form of thyroid disease and most of them are women. However, most of them were mildly hypothyroid. As in other studies in developed countries, hypothyroidism tends to increase with age and is more common in women, and people with goitre. A study reported that hypothyroidism was more prevalent (40.5%) in the age group of 36-45 years with obvious female preponderance (Haddow *et al.*, 1999). It is also reported that maternal hypothyroidism and hypothyroxemia occurring in the first half of pregnancy might be harmful to embryo foetal brain development and lead to intellectual retardation in the offspring (Pop, *et al.*, 2003).

Women have 10 times the risk of hypothyroidism as compared to men, with the difference being significant after age 34. Because the symptoms of hypothyroidism and menopause are so similar, hypothyroidism may easily be missed. Pregnancy is a major factor in the higher risk in women. It affects the thyroid in a number of ways and poses a high risk for hypothyroidism, both during pregnancy and afterward. For one, iodine requirements are high in both the mother and the foetus. Changes in reproductive hormones also cause changes in thyroid hormone levels. In addition, some women develop antibodies to their own thyroid during pregnancy, causing a condition known as postpartum auto-immune, or sub-acute thyroiditis. This occurs in up to 10 per cent of pregnant women and tends to develop 4-12 months after delivery. It is a limited condition and nearly always clears up. However, it does pose a risk for the development of permanent hypothyroidism later on. The risk for hypothyroidism is greatest after age 50 and increases with age. However, hypothyroidism can affect people of all ages.

Thyroid disorders are one of the most commonly encountered endocrine disorders in India. It is estimated that there are at least 42 million individual with thyroid disorders in India and the effect it has on the women of reproductive age is noteworthy. A study from Mumbai have suggested that congenital hypothyroidism is common in India, incidence being 1 out of 2640 neonates whereas worldwide frequency is 1 in 4000 live births and is associated with significant neurological and development morbidity, much of which can be prevented by early diagnosis and treatment (Choudhury, 2012). In India amongst adult population, the prevalence of hypothyroidism is recently studied in Cochin. Amongst 971 adult subjects, the prevalence of hypothyroidism was 3.9 per cent. The prevalence of subclinical hypothyroidism was more being 9.4 per cent. In women the prevalence was higher, at 11.4 per cent, when compared with man, in whom the prevalence was 6.2 per cent (Unnikrishnan and Menon, 2011).

Hypothyroidism in North East Indian Population

As mentioned above, North East India being located in the foothills of Himalayas is considered to be in the classical goitreendemic belt of India, this is extremely significant in view of the fact that iodine deficiency is one of the risk factors of congenital hypothyroidism (Singh *et al.*, 2013). So far, a few epidemiological surveys have been conducted to study the prevalence of hypothyroidism in the population inhabiting the foothills of the Himalayas (Terai region) and Assam only, where the prevalence of hypothyroidism has been reported to be very high (Teinhoven *et al.*, 2015) (Table 6.1).

In North East India out of 2456 randomly analysed blood samples over a period of one year hypothyroidism is being high with a prevalence of 10.9 per cent and sub-clinical hypothyroidism being 13.1 per cent (Choudhury, 2012). In another study on prevalence of hypothyroidism in women of reproductive age in Meghalaya, North

Table 6.1: Studies on Hypothyroidism in North East India

States	*Study design*	*Key Findings*	*References*
Assam	Randomly analysed blood samples (hospital based studies)	Hypothyroidism is 10.9 per cent, sub Clinical Hypothyroidism is 13.1 per cent	Choudhury, 2012
Manipur	Retrospective study conducted at RIMS among 500 cases during 5 yrs	38.4 per cent had thyroid disorders, 45.55 per cent of female had hyperthyroidism, 43.35 per cent of female had hypothyroidism, 6.11 per cent of female had sub clinical hypothyroidism, 4.44 per cent of female had overt hypothyroidism	Jebasingh, *et al.*, 2015
	A study conducted on 400 1st and 2nd trimester pregnant women in the Department of Obstetrics and Gynaecology, JNIMS, Imphal	18 per cent of them have sub- clinical hypothyroidism and 4.5 per cent have overt hypothyroidism.	Singh *et al.*, 2015
Meghalaya	A study on 90 non-pregnant women and 70 pregnant women of Meghalaya, between the Age group of 15-25 years and 36-45 years age group.	3.33 per cent of hypothyroidism in non-pregnant women of 36-45 yrs, 3.70 per cent of hypothyroidism in pregnant women of 15-25 yrs.	Kharkongor and Gupta, 1998

Source: Author's Study.

Eastern India recorded 3.33 per cent prevalence of hypothyroidism in non-pregnant women of 36-45 years age group and 3.70 per cent prevalence of hypothyroidism in pregnant women of 15-25 years age group. Since hypothyroidism was found in individual belonging to 15-25 years age group and 36-45 years age group, ideally pregnancy should be avoided during the early and late years of reproductive age of women. When considering the total number of samples, 1.11 per cent prevalence of hypothyroidism was recorded among non-pregnant women and 1.43 per cent prevalence of hypothyroidism was recorded among pregnant women (Kharkongor and Gupta, 1998).

Very few studies have come up from Manipur, as per the published data. A study conducted by (Das *et al.*, 2013) states that hypothyroidism is among the most common endocrine disorder encountered during pregnancy and reproductive age group. Endemic iodine deficiency and autoimmune disease remain a major cause of hypothyroidism. In their study on the prevalence of Hypothyroidism among pregnant women in the Sub-mountain State of Manipur, they recruited 400 1st and 2nd trimester pregnant women who were registered in the Department of Obstetrics and Gynaecology, Jawaharlal Nehru Institution of Medical Sciences, Imphal (Singh *et al.*, 2015), reported higher prevalence of hypothyroidism especially of SCH among these women.

A retrospective study conducted at RIMS among 500 cases during 5 yrs of studies have shown that 38.4 per cent had thyroid disorders, 45.55 per cent of female had hyperthyroidism, 43.35 per cent of female had hypothyroidism, 6.11 per cent of female had sub-clinical hypothyroidism, 4.44 per cent of female had overt hypothyroidism (Jebasingh *et al.*, 2015). According to Demitrost and Ranabir (2012) approximately 1 in 10 adult female gender and old age were found to have significant association with hypothyroidism.

Hypothyroidism and its Association with Other Diseases

Iodine has important effects on human health and social development and its deficiency constitutes one of the major international public health problems (Alexander *et al.*, 2011). Iodine in adequate amounts (RDA:150 μg) is a prerequisite for the biosynthesis of thyroid hormones (TH) by the thyroid gland. In case of deficiency of dietary iodine, the rate of TH biosynthesis is decreased resulting in a condition called hypothyroidism. Continued lack of iodine in the diet leads to iodine deficiency disorders (IDD) like goitre (clinical hypothyroidism) and endemic cretinism associated with mental retardation, deafness and ataxia, lower IQ etc. (Dhanwal *et al.*, 2013). Hypothyroidism during foetal/post-natal life interferes with the normal development and maturation of the central nervous system (Demitrost and Ranabir, 2012, Das *et al.*, 2013) and increases the chances of infant mortality, congenital abnormalities, stunted growth and dwarfism associated with a waddling gait etc. (Aronson, 2008; Das *et al.*, 2013). Hypothyroidism during childhood results in impaired mental functions and psychology (Demitrost and Ranabir, 2012; Singh *et al.*, 2013). Further, in hypothyroidic individuals sexual maturation and the onset of puberty is also delayed. In adults, hypothyroidism is associated with reduced fertility, impaired mental function (American Thyroid Association, 2011), coronary heart diseases and atherosclerosis, anaemia (Ahmad *et al.*, 2013), pleural effusions of the respiratory system, reduced appetite, constipation, delayed muscle contraction and relaxation, decreased renal blood flow and glomerular filtration rate etc. In pregnant women hypothyroidism leads to abortion and premature delivery, still birth or birth of congenitally defective babies (Pop *et al.*, 2003; Green *et al.*, 2011; Geffari *et al.*, 2013).

Studies have also found that thyroid dysfunction is much common in diabetic population compared to non-diabetic population, and diabetes and thyroid disorders have been shown to mutually influence each other (Bharat *et al.*, 2013). Most often thyroid dysfunction and type 1 diabetes are due to an autoimmune condition, whereas type 2 diabetes is mainly due to insulin resistance (Geffari *et al.*, 2013). Thus, it seems that diabetes, especially type 1, has potential link with thyroid dysfunction or *vice versa*. Besides the effects due to high blood glucose in diabetics, low thyroid hormones independently increase the risk for cardiovascular diseases in both diabetic and non-diabetic patients (Aronson, 2008). People with many autoimmune diseases have a higher risk for hypothyroidism. Type 1 (insulin-dependent) diabetes poses a higher risk and is a special problem since hypothyroidism can affect insulin requirements. Diabetic patients have a higher prevalence of thyroid disorders compared with the general population, because patients with one organ specific autoimmune disease are at risk of developing other autoimmune disorders (Umpierrez *et al.*, 2003; Wu, 2008). A number of reports have, however, indicated a higher than normal prevalence of thyroid disorders in type 2 diabetic patients, with hypothyroidism being the most common disorder (Nobre *et al.*, 2002). In other studies the frequency of hypothyroidism in patients with diabetes mellitus has been reported as 0.7 per cent to 4 per cent and hyperthyroidism has varied from 3.2 per cent to 4.6 per cent (Sugreene, *et al.*, 1982). The physiological and biochemical inter-relationship between Insulin and iodothyronines and the influence of both insulin and iodothyronines on the metabolism of carbohydrates, proteins and lipids are recorded (Sugreene *et al.*, 1982; Mayne, 1998). The presence of thyroid dysfunction may affect diabetes control.

Smoking significantly increases risk for thyroid disease, particularly autoimmune Hashimoto's thyroiditis and postpartum thyroiditis. Smoking also increases the negative effects of hypothyroidism, notably on the arteries and heart. People with certain medical conditions have a higher risk for hypothyroidism. These conditions include autoimmune diseases. Women with other autoimmune diseases, including systemic lupus erythematosus, pernicious anaemia, and rheumatoid arthritis, are also at higher risk for hypothyroidism. Pregnant women with autoimmune conditions have a 25 per cent risk for hypothyroidism during gestation. Hypothyroidism and gout often coexist and may have biologic mechanisms in common. People with eating disorders are at risk for hypothyroidism. In these patients, however, reduced thyroid function may be an adaptation to malnutrition and, therefore, some experts think that only the eating disorder should be treated, not hypothyroidism. As many as half of patients with Turner syndrome have hypothyroidism, usually in the form of Hashimoto's thyroiditis. This inherited condition is one of the most common genetic diseases in women. Many drugs affect the thyroid, so anyone being treated for a chronic disease, taking thyroid medication, and those at risk for a thyroid disorder should discuss the impact these drugs may have on their thyroid.

Therefore, keeping in view the severe adverse effects of TH deficiency among the general population, particularly in women and the lack of information about the status of the hypothyroidism in the North East region of India, there is potential of unreported or undiagnosed case of thyroid hormone dysfunction in the general population of North East India, which become significant under the approach of translational research, reaching out to masses. North East India being a hilly states in the South East Asian region, where there is risk of thyroid dysfunction particularly hypothyroidism, the underreported prevalence is also expected. A few studies, have come from Hospital or restricted to only the patients. Therefore, screening of thyroid hormones dysfunction in the general population beyond the hospital based study will be the prerequisite in the present days as such underreport would affect the morbidity of the general population.

Conclusion

Hypothyroidism is a common endocrine disorder having multiple etiology. Early diagnosis and treatment are essential to prevent irreversible and permanent nervous system damage and developmental delay. Therefore, screening of risk factors, timely diagnosis and treatment are essential for diagnosing the prevalence of hypothyroidism that will help future researches in their studies to help the general populations.

References

Al-Geffari, M., Ahmad, N.A., Al-Sharqawi, A. H., Youssef, A.M., Alnaqeb, D., Al-Rubeaan, K. (2013). "Risk factors for thyroid dysfunction among type 2 diabetic patients in a highly diabetes mellitus prevalent society", *International Journal of Endocrinology*, Vol. 2013, Article ID 417920, 6 pages, 2013.

American Diabetes Association (2015). "Classification and diagnosis of diabetes", *Diabetes Care,* 38(1): S8-S16.

Aronson, D. (2008). Hyperglycemia and the pathobiology of diabetic complications, *Advances in Cardiology,* 45:1-16.

Bashir, M.I., Wani, A.I., Bhat, M.H., Sheikh, M.I., Ganie, M.A., Zargar, A.H. (2004). Profile of Thyroid Disorders in Kashmir valley *Journal of Endocrinology and Metabolism,* 6: 32-35.

Bharat, Hijam, D., Gangte, D., Lalnunpui, Premchand, Devi, I. and Singh, Gyaneshwar, W. (2013). "Mellitus Thyroid Status in Diabetes", *J Glycomics Lipidomics,* 3:106.

Das, A., Shaini, L., Sangeeta, N., Saurav, P., Chanchal, L., Singh S.D. and Ahilya, P. (2013). "Prevalence of Thyroid Hormone Dysfunction among Female Patients, Attending a Multispeciality Hospital in Manipur", *IOSR Journal of Dental and Medical Sciences,* 10(2): 7-11.

Demitrost, L. and Ranabir S. (2012). "Thyroid dysfunction in type 2 diabetes mellitus. A retrospective study", *Indian J. Endocrinol Metab.,* 16 (Suppl. 2): S334-5.

Dhanwal, D.K., Prasad, S., Agrawal, A.K., Dixit, V. and Banerjee, A.K. (2013). "High prevalence of subclinical hypothyroidism during first trimester of pregnancy in North India", *Indian J. Endocrinol Metab.,* 17:281-4.

Haddow, J.E., Palomaki, G.E., Allan, W.C., Williams, J.R., Knight, G.T., Gagnon, J., O'Heir, C.E., Mitchel, M.L., Rosalie, J., Waisbren, S.E., Faix, J.D., Klein, R.Z. (1999). "Maternal Thyroid Deficiency during Pregnancy and Subsequent Neuropsychological Development of the Child", *N Engl. J. Med.,* 341:549-555.

Hollowell, J.G., Steahling, M.W., Flanders, W.D., Hannon, W.H., Gunter, E.W., Spencer C.A., Braveman, L.E. (2002). "Serum TSH, T4 and Thyroid antibodies in United States population (1988-1994): National Health and Nutrition Examination Survey (NHANES III)", *J. Clin. Endocrinol. Metal.*, 87: 489-499.

Jebasingh, F.K., Salam, R., Meetei, T.L., Singh, N.N., Prasad, L. (2015). "Thyroid status of the pregnant women of Manipur: A comparison of American Thyroid Association guidelines and normal laboratory reference range", *Thyroid Res Pract.,* 12:67-70.

Kharkongor, I.J. and Gupta, B.B.P. (1998). "Study on prevalence of hypothyroidism in women of reproductive age in Meghalaya, North Eastern India", *Current Science,* 75(12):1390-1393.

Lewis, E. Braveman and Robert, D. Utiger (2005). "Introduction to hypothyroidism", *The Thyroid: A Fundamental and Clinical Text, Ninth Edition* (Lippincott Wiliams and Wilkins), 9: 697-699.

Mayne, P.D., Mayne, P. and Day, A. (1998). Carbohydrate metabolism. In: *Clinical Chemistry in Diagnosis and Treatment,* 6th Edition (Hodder Arnold Publication) Glasgow, Barth: Colourbooks, pp. 195-222.

Medhuri Devdhar, Yasser H. Ousman Kenneth D. Burman (2007). Hyothyroidism. *Endocrinology and Metabolic Clinics of North America,* 36:5-93.

Michael, T., Dermott, M.C. and Ridgway, E.C. (2009). "Hypothyroidism", In: Cooper, D.S. (Ed.), *Medical Management of Thyroid Diseases*, New York: Informa Healthcare, pp. 145-179.

Niafar, M., Aliasgharzadeh, A., Bahrami, A. and Najafipur, F. (2009). "Prevalence of thyroid dysfunction in the elderly women of Iran", *Endocrine Abstracts,* 20: 137.

Nobre, E.L., Jorge, Z., Pratas, S., Silva, C. and Castro, J.J. (2002). "Profile of the thyroid function in a population with type-2 diabetes mellitus", *Endocrine Abstracts*, 3:298.

Perros, P., McCrimmon, R.J., Shaw, G. and Frier, B.M. (1995). "Frequency of thyroid dysfunction in diabetic patients: value of annual screening", *Diabetic Medicine*, 12: 622-7.

Pop, V.J., Brouwers, E.P., Vader, H.L., Vulsma, T., van Baar A.L., deVijlder, J.J. (2003). "Maternal hypothyroxinaemia during early pregnancy and subsequent child development: a 3-year follow-up study", *Clinical Endocrinology,* 59 (3):282-88.

Singh, R.A., Devi, K.G., Devi, K.L., Banik, U. (2013). "New-born screening for congenital hypothyroidism in Manipur by measurement of umbilical cord thyroid stimulating hormone: A hospital based study", *J. Med. Soc.,* 27:127-30

Stagnaro-Green, A., Abalovich, M., Alexander, E., Azizi, F., Mestman, J., Negro, R., Nixon, A., Pearce, E.N., Soldin, O.P., Sullivan, S. and Wiersinga, W. (2011). *Guidelines of the American Thyroid Association for the diagnosis and management of thyroid disease during pregnancy and postpartum Thyroid*, 21:108-125.

Sugreene, D.D., McEnvoy, M., Drury, M.I. (1982). "Thyroid disease in diabetes", *Postgrad Med. J.,* 58(865): 680-684.

Umpierrez, G.E., Latif, K.A., Murphy, M.B., Lambcth, H.C., Stentz, F., Bush, A., Kitabchi, A.E. (2003). "Thyroid dysfunction in patients with type 1 diabetes: a longitudinal study", *Diabetes Care,* 26(4):1181-1185.

Unnikrishnon, A.G. and Menon, U.V. (2011). "Thyroid Disorders in India: An epidemiological perspective", *Indian J. of Endocrinology and Metabolism,* 15 (2): 78-81.

Usha, M.V., Sundaram, K.R., Unnikrishnan, A.G., Jayakumar, R.V., Nair, V., Kumar, H. (2009). "High prevalence of undetected thyroid disorders in an iodine sufficient adult south Indian population", *J. Indian Med. Assoc.*, 107:72 7.

Van Tienhoven-Wind L.J.N. and Dullaart, R.P.F. (2015), Low-normal thyroid function and novel cardiometabolic biomarkers, *Nutrients,* 7(2):1352-1377.

Wu, P. (2008). "Thyroid Disease and Diabetes", *Clinical Diabetes,* 18(1):38.

7

Incidence of Type 2 Diabetes among the Physically Active and Inactive Population of Manipur

Ksh. BeliyaLuxmi Devi and *S. Jibonkumar Singh*

Introduction

Human lifestyle is changing tremendously day by day as an outcome of rapid advancement in the field of science and technology. People are enjoying and preferring 'push button' way of life to tiresome physically active way of earning livelihood. This preference and changing life style to comfort living spending less time in physical activities have resulted to more inactiveness in every ways. The consequence of physically inactiveness of our body leads to different life style diseases. Diabetes is one such disease among others which is life threatening and chronic. Diabetes is a group of metabolic diseases characterized by hyperglycaemia resulting from defects in insulin secretion, insulin action, or both. The chronic hyperglycaemia of diabetes is associated with long-term damage, dysfunction, and failure of different organs, especially the eyes, kidneys, nerves, heart, and blood vessels (American Diabetes Association, 2010). Diabetes can be of types in general they are Type 1 diabetes (T1D) and Type 2 diabetes (T2D). Type 1 diabetes case, formerly called juvenile-onset or insulin-dependent diabetes, is rare and it accounts for 5 to 10 out of 100 people who have diabetes. Diabetes may be caused by different factors while environment or life style plays great role, however, almost 50 per cent of the Diabetic patients have one of the parents or family members affected with the disease. Till now the genes responsible have not been isolated but a strong correlation exists. Stress of our life like frequent quarrelling, live threatening, work pressure etc. also found to be strongly related with diabetes due to the released hormones called adrenaline and cortisol, (Dr. Chhajer, 2009). Both of them have tremendous capacity to increase blood glucose. According to "National Population Health Surveys" of Canada (Katzmarzyk, 2008), being sedentary or physically inactive means expending less than 1.5 kcal/kg/day energy in leisure physical activities. This is the equivalent of walking a little over two kilometres or 1.3 miles, or approximately 3000 steps. For most people, that is a walk of 25 minutes or less. Physically active, therefore, refers to those persons who, professionally or as a way of life, do works more than 25 minutes for the requirement or the substitution of their physical activities. For example, unskilled labourers, cultivators, carpenters, masons, and sportsmen, etc. On the contrary, the Inactive persons are those whose works are more of mental activity rather than physical activities. These groups are confronted with a number of lifestyle diseases and health problem due to the accumulation of more amount of adipose tissue resulting to obese condition. For example, diabetes mellitus is known to have genetic component but environmental factors like dietary habit and lifestyles of the persons play an important role in the penetrance and expressivity of the gene. In general, physically active person are physically fit and less prone to life style diseases as compared to inactive persons. Anthropometric studies have shown that the pattern of body fat distribution is an important risk factor for coronary heart disease (CHD), non-insulin dependent diabetes (NIDDM) and hypertension (Das *et al.*, 2000). Concerning with diabetes mellitus, it is caused by deficiency of insulin hormone due to hypoactivity of β-cells of Islet of Langerhans of pancreases, obesity and over weightiness, mental shocks and heredity. NIDDM or Type 2 occurs due to the failure of the target cells to take up insulin from the blood. The history of the beginning of the study of this disease dates back to 2000 years ago in Egypt and in ancient Indian Ayurveda by Indian physician (Shah, 2000). Type-2 diabetes is produced by both genetic and environmental factors. It is learnt from the study that genes are thought to play major role in the etiology of type 2 diabetes (Ghattu *et al.*, 2005). On the other hand, sedentary life style is considered as a main risk factor for DM-II (Esteghamati *et al.*, 2008). In a similar approach, avoidance of adiposity by enhanced physical activity and regulated calorie intake can be measured to prevent and control diabetes epidemic (Rajeev *et al.*,

2007). Increasing risk of Type 2 diabetes due to increased prevalence of overweight and obesity as a consequence of modernization and less physical activities is experienced in China (Raquel *et al.*, 2006). One of the study indicates that diabetic female have higher mean values for endomorphy and mesomorphy and lesser mean value for ectomorphy than their males counterpart. The level of physical activity either is the key factor to control or enhanced the diseases (Vikram *et al.*, 2007). On the other hand, another finding reveals that total height was weakly and inversely associated with diabetes to mask the differences in the association with leg and trunk length (Lawlor *et al.*, 2002). Among the anthropometric parameters, Waist Circumference is a better predictor than is WHR (Youfa *et al.*, 2005). In another study, large hip and thigh circumference are associated with a lower risk of type 2 diabetes, independently of BMI, age, and waist circumference, whereas a large waist circumference is associated with a higher risk. Similarly, it is also mentioned that both overall and abdominal adiposity strongly and independently predict risk of type 2 diabetes (Meisinger *et al.*, 2006). According to one of the recent findings, Caucasian women with gestational diabetes mellitus (GDM) are shorter than pregnant women without GDM regardless of the diagnostic criteria used or the severity of glucose intolerance (Jaroslaw *et al.*, 2010).

A study of diabetes and its treatment with special reference to Bengalese and their diet conducted by Chakravarthy in the year 1938 may probably be the first systematic study on the prevalence of diabetes in India. Though a number of studies relating to the relationship of Type II DM and physique had so far been conducted among different population groups of India, no such studies have ever been conducted among the population groups of Manipur. Keeping this in view, and considering the importance of the work from the health point of view of the people, the present work aims to examine the risk of type II DM among the Physically Active (PA) and Inactive (IA) population of Manipur from an anthropological perspective.

Materials and Method

The present study which attempts to study the blood sugar level and BMI status among the Physically Active and Inactive population was conducted in Manipur—one of the North—eastern states of India. According to National Population Health Surveys of Canada (2005), those who expend less than 1.5 kcal/kg of energy per day in leisure physical activities which is almost equivalent of walking a little over two kilometres or 1.3 miles, or approximately 3000 steps in 25 minutes or less are considered as sedentary or physically inactive people. On the other hand, those persons who, professionally or as a way of life, do works more than 25 minutes for the requirement or the substitution of their physical activities are considered as physically active person. Data for the present study was collected from a total of 429 randomly selected samples representing Meitei population of Bishnupur district, Manipur, whose age range between 20 to 70 years. The sample comprised 200 males (96 Physically Active, 104 Inactive) and 219 females (107 Physically Active and 112 Inactive). Physically active population are collected from rural area and inactive from the urban area. Two important body measurements, i.e. body weight and body height, were taken for calculation of BMI. To examine the cases of diabetes a biochemical test was conducted by using Accu-Chek Active Monitor which measured blood glucose for the detection of Type 2 Diabetes. For classifying BMI, the WHO classification of BMI was used (WHO, 2010). The data were exposed to appropriate statistical treatments for a systematic analysis and meaningful interpretation.

Results and Discussion

Based on the present findings it is observed that, the blood glucose content increases with increasing chronological age in both the sexes irrespective of either PA or IA group (Tables 7.1 and 7.2). This finding is, therefore, in agreement with the earlier findings of different scholars (Sullivam *et al.*, 1974) and (Gary *et al.*, 2006). It is also clearly evident that Inactive subject of both sexes have higher mean value of blood glucose content than physically active subjects. Similar findings wherein the chances of having diabetes and diabetes-related cardiovascular comorbidities increased with BMI regardless of physical activity and increased with physical inactivity regardless of BMI (Sullivan *et al.*, 2005). Among the IA group highest blood glucose content is observed in the age group 60-70 years for both the genders (Male–166.00±2.02 mg/dl; Females–132.00±2.38 mg/dl). Among the PA group, males belonging to age group 40–50 years

Table 7.1: Random Blood Glucose Status of Physical Active (PA) and Inactive (IA) Meitei Males of Manipur

Age range (in yrs.)	*Class*	*f*	*%*	χ^2 *(mg/dl)*	*SD*	*t-test*
20–30	PA	18	9.00	91.83±1.25	5.32	0.10
	IA	22	11.00	92.00±1.14	5.36	
30–40	PA	21	10.50	93.12±0.82	3.74	17.49*
	IA	24	12.00	119.17±1.25	6.16	
40–50	PA	19	9.50	127.15±1.02	4.46	13.72*
	IA	24	12.00	156.92±1.92	9.43	
50–60	PA	20	10.00	105.58±1.16	5.21	30.30*
	IA	18	9.00	138.61±1.60	6.80	
60–70	PA	18	9.00	112.50±1.25	5.31	22.48*
	IA	16	8.00	166.00±2.02	8.09	
Total	**PA**	**96**	**48.00**	**106.16±1.71**	**16.78**	**11.20***
	IA	**104**	**52.00**	**134.04±1.81**	**18.46**	

Source: Author's Study.

Table 7.2: Random Blood Glucose Status of Physical Active (PA) and Inactive (IA) Meitei Females of Manipur

Age ranges	*Class*	*f*	*%*	χ^2 *(mg/dl)*	*SD*	*t-value*
20–30	PA	12	5.48	84.92±2.82	9.78	0.02
	IA	19	8.68	85.00±2.40	10.48	
30–40	PA	34	15.53	94.79±1.83	10.67	5.58*
	IA	32	14.61	108.69±1.69	9.58	
40–50	PA	23	10.50	109.48±1.68	8.08	0.60
	IA	21	9.59	107.52±2.79	12.78	
50–60	PA	21	9.59	101.20±3.03	9.57	3.46*
	IA	25	13.23	113.96±2.09	11.63	
60–70	PA	17	7.76	118.80±2.15	8.87	4.44*
	IA	15	6.84	132.00±2.38	9.23	
Total	**PA**	**107**	**48.86**	**102.05±1.51**	**15.62**	
	IA	**112**	**51.14**	**109.72±1.62**	**17.19**	**3.45***

Source: Author's Study.

have highest blood glucose level (127.15±1.02 mg/dl) in contrast to that of females among whom the highest (118.80±2.15 mg/dl) is seen in the age group 60–70 years. Coming to the lowest blood glucose content, both PA and IA group of either of the sexes belonging to 20–30 years of age group display the lowest value (Male–PA

91.83±1.25 mg/dl, IA 92.00±1.14 mg/dl; Female—PA 84.92±2, 82 mg/dl, IA 85.00±2.40 mg/dl) respectively.

One of the common feature observed in the distribution of sugar level content in different age groups among the PA and IA males is that, all the age groups except 20-30 years show significant difference (*see* t-value, Table 7.1). While looking into the overall mean sugar level of male population, IA group is found to have higher mean value (134.04±1.81 mg/dl) that PA group (106.16±1.71 mg/dl), thereby showing statistically significant difference (t = 11.20, Table 7.1). The difference observed in the blood sugar level between PA and IA may obviously be because of burning more calories as a result of exposure to physical activity and manual labour among the rural populations. Similarly, among the females too excepting the age group 20–30 years and 40–50 years, IA group of other age groups have higher blood sugar level than the PA groups. Again on the whole IA females have higher blood sugar level (109.72±1.62 mg/dl) than the PA females (102.05±1.51 mg/dl) showing a statistical significant difference (t = 3.45, Table 7.2).

Table 7.3 displays the distribution pattern of Risk of Type 2 Diabetes (R), Type 2 Diabetes (D) and Normal (N) among PA and IA male population in relation to BMI status. It is clearly evident from the table that highest frequency per cent of both the population belong to normal BMI level though PA group is higher (87.50%)

Table 7.3: Frequency distribution of Risk of Type 2 Diabetes (R), Type 2 Diabetes (D) and Normal (N) by BMI for Male

BMI (kg/m2)	*Class*	*R*	*%*	*D*	*%*	*N*	*%*	*Total*	*d*
								f	*%*
Underweight	PA			1	0.96	10	10.42	11	11.46
	IA					2	1.92	2	1.92
Normal	PA			2	2.08	52	54.17	54	56.25
	IA	2	1.92	11	10.58	29	27.88	42	40.38
Overweight	PA	4	4.17	5	5.21	22	22.92	31	32.29
	IA	15	14.42	9	8.65	25	24.04	49	47.12
Obese	IA			4	3.85	5	4.81	9	8.65
Obese class II	IA					2	1.92	2	1.92
Total	**PA**	**4**	**4.17**	**8**	**8.34**	**84**	**87.50**	**96**	**100**
	IA	**17**	**16.35**	**24**	**23.08**	**63**	**60.58**	**104**	**100**

Source: Author's Study.

than the IA group (60.58%). It is also observed that IA group has higher frequency of Risk of Type 2 Diabetes (16.35%), Type 2 Diabetes (23.08%) individuals than PA group who have 4.17 per cent and 8.34 per cent respectively. Considering the BMI status of the population it is evident that among the Physically Active and Inactive males the highest frequency is observed for normal BMI range (physically active–54.17% and inactive-27.88%). When we consider the Diabetic category highest frequency of Inactive population belong to Normal BMI (10.58%) followed by overweight category (8.65%) and obese class I (3.85%). As for females (Table 7.4) highest frequency per cent of both PA group (89.42%) and IA group (75.89%) have normal sugar level with 56.73% PA and 33.04 per cent IA belonging to the category of Normal BMI status.

Table 7.4: Frequency Distribution of Risk of Type 2 Diabetes (R), Type 2 Diabetes (D) and Normal (N) by BMI for Female

BMI	*Class*	*R*	*%*	*D*	*%*	*N*	*%*	*Total*	
								f	*%*
Underweight	PA					14	13.46	14	13.46
	IA			4	3.57	9	8.04	13	11.61
Normal range	PA	2	1.92	3	2.88	59	56.73	64	61.54
	IA	2	1.79	8	7.14	37	33.04	47	41.96
Overweight	PA	2	1.92	4	3.84	20	19.23	26	25.00
	IA	3	2.68	10	8.93	31	27.68	44	39.29
Obese	IA					7	6.25	7	6.25
Obese class II	IA					1	0.99	1	0.99
Total	**PA**	**4**	**3.84**	**7**	**6.73**	**93**	**89.42**	**104**	**100**
	IA	**5**	**4.46**	**22**	**19.64**	**85**	**75.89**	**112**	**100**

Source: Author's Study.

As many as 8.93 per cent of the total female population belonging to inactive group have overweight category of BMI in contrast to 3.84 per cent of IA Group. Inactive individuals (7.14%) and PA (2.88%) who belong to normal BMI range are also reported to have diabetes. It is revealed that as many as 3.84 per cent of PA and 4.84 per cent of IA are found to have risk for Type 2 diabetes in present study.

Overall findings of the present study reveal that physically inactive subject of almost all age groups of both sexes have higher mean value of blood glucose content than physically active subjects. It is also observed that physical activities are much more reduced in urban areas as compared to rural areas. Similar studies also reports that Physical activity is significantly lower and differs in pattern in urban subjects compared to rural. Physical inactivity is associated with these diseases, although not always significant in women (Esobngwi, 2002). On comparing the socio-economic status, physically active group being from rural population have lower socio-economic status and thus exposed to more manual work for their livelihood. As a result they have lower blood glucose level than their counterparts of urban population. This finding is in consistency with that of Ramachandran *et al.*, (2002), who reported that the prevalence of diabetes was lower in the low living socio-economic group (12.6 *vs*. 24.6%) due to the relative degree of their physical activity. The present findings and results are also supported by the study of Raquel *et al.*, (2006), who studied Shangai women population of China, Rajeev *et al.*, (2007) studied and examined the regional disparity of diabetes among Indian population and Esteghamati *et al.*, (2008) work on Iran. As compared to male counterparts females have lesser degree of significant difference in the distribution pattern of blood sugar level between PA and IA. This may be because of the fact that women in urban area, even though, are not manual workers, they are more involved in day-to-day household activities which amounts to some degree of physical activities as compared to the male counterparts of IA males. In line with the present study Esobngwi (2002) reported that diabetes was more prevalent in urban compared to rural women ($P<0.05$), but not men. Urban subjects were characterized by lower physical activity ($P<0.001$), light occupation, high prevalence of multiple occupations, and reduced walking and cycling time compared to rural subjects. Increasing physical activity is associated with a significant reduction in risk for diabetes, whereas a sedentary life-style is directly related to risk (Frank *et al.*, 2001).

The findings of the present study also reveal that the Risk of Type 2 Diabetes (R) and incidence of Type 2 Diabetes (D) increase with increasing BMI and obesity status in both the sexes though with a higher frequency among the inactive population. This finding is also in agreement with some of the earlier reports which says that Obesity and physical inactivity are well-established risk factors for the development of Type 2 diabetes (Franz, 2002; Klein, 2004; American Diabetes Association, 2003; U.S. Department of Health and Human Services, 2001 and 2005). Again as evidenced from the study those with lower BMI are more engaged in physical activities and less risk for diabetes and less prevalence of diabetes. Similar findings were also reported by Sullivan *et al.,* 2005, who worked among the US population.

Review of literature says that today profile of disease pattern is gradually changing from infectious disease and nutritional deficiency diseases to life style diseases (WHO, 2008) which accounts to more than 60 per cent global death (WHO, 2014). And it is expected that by 2020 it will account for 69 per cent of global death in developing countries, and a major cause of death in the world by 2030 (Sacco *et al.*, 2013). And as for prevalence of diabetes is concerned it will almost double in the next 25 years and at least 75 per cent will be in developing countries (Pongen, 2017). Considering Indian population, it has been reported that 19.3 million Indians were diagnosed with diabetes mellitus in 1995 and will surpass 57.2 million by 2025 (Deedawania and Singh, 2005).

In short life style diseases including diabetes are becoming a public health issue of the contemporary human society and timely address and intervention is the urgent need. For this different strategies for combating diabetes needs to be implemented at different levels more particularly in urban areas where people are physically in active. Government should take up necessary steps to address the issue well in time before it is too late.

The present study is simply based on only three parameters, i.e. body height and body weight for assessment of body mass index, and blood sugar level for assessment of status of risk for type 2 diabetes and prevalence of type 2 diabetes. Though the findings can reveal some of the general inference, there is a need for further in depth study incorporating some other physiological parameters like blood pressure, pulse rate, waist hip ratio, body fat composition and somatotyping for providing an overall comparative evaluation between physically active and inactive population of the said community.

Conclusion

The change in life style to sedentary, people becomes more inactive in every ways. They go for comfort living and spend less time in physical activities, most of the people and still not aware of what affects them in shifting life style. With physically inactiveness our body is more prone to different diseases such as Diabetes, Obesity, Coronary Heart disease, Blood pressure etc. and some of the diseases are life threatening and chronic. Owing to different environmental exposure the two groups of people, i.e. Physically Active (PA) and Inactive (IA) population are naturally expected to have number of variation in physique, health condition. In general, physically active persons are physically fit and less prone to life style diseases as compared to inactive peer group in both the gender. Type 2 Diabetes is known to have genetic factor but environmental components like dietary habit and life style of the persons play an important role in the penetrance and expressivity of the gene. Findings of the present study reveals that blood glucose level increases with increase of chronological age and physically active persons irrespective of sex have more prevalence of overweight and obese condition and are more prone to develop Type 2 diabetes and also risk for Type 2 diabetes. To keep body, mind in balance and free from diseases for a sound healthy country, 'Physically Activeness' is the sacred medicine for human health.

Acknowledgements

We extend our heartily thanks to all the participants for their tremendous cooperation and warm hospitality during our data collection. We are extremely thankful to our friends for the help they provided to us during our field programme. We shall always remain thankful to them.

References

American Diabetes Association (2003). "National Institute of Diabetes, Digestive and Kidney Diseases: The prevention or delay of Type 2 diabetes (Position Statement)", *Diabetes Care* 26 (Suppl. 1): S62-S69.

American Diabetes Association, Arlington, Verginia, US. (2010). "Definition and description of diabetes mellitus", *Diabetes Care,* 33 (Suppl-1) S62-S69.

Chakravarthy, A. (1938). "A study of diabetes and its treatment with special reference to Bengales and their diet", *Indian Med. Rec.*, 56-58.

Chhajer (2009). *Cure Diabetes*, New Delhi: Diamond Pocket Book (P) Ltd. Fusion Books.

Das Choudhury, A.B. and K. Bose (2000). "A review of studies on central body fat distribution among Indians", In: *Discovery of North East India, 6,* Kolkata: Salmoli Publication, pp. 1-10.

Deedwania, P. and Singh, V. (2005). "Coronary artery disease in South Asians: Evolving strategies for treatment and prevention. *Indian Heart J.,* 57(6): 617 31.

Dutta, Arindam, Santa Naorem, Singh Premchand, Th. (2005). "Prevalence of peripheral neuropathy in newly diagnosed type 2 diabetics", *Int. J.Diab. Dev. Countries,* 25:30-33.

Esteghamati, A., Hassabi, M., Halabchi, F., and Bagheri, M. (2008). "Exercise prescription in patients with diabetes type 2", *Ind. J. Dia. and Lipid Disorder,* 8:1-15.

Frank B. Hu, M.D.; Michael F. Leitzmann, M.D.; Meir L. Stampfer, M.D.; Graham A. Colditz, M.D.; Walter C. Willett, M.D., and Eric B. Rimm, ScD. (2001). "Physical activity and television watching in relation to risk for type 2 diabetes mellitus in men", *Arch. Intern. Med.,* 161:1542-1548.

Franz, M.J., Bantle, J.P., Beebe, C.A., Brunzell, J.D., Chiasson, J.L., Garg, A., Holzmeister, L.A., Hoogwerf, B., Mayer-Davis, E., Mooradian, A.D., Purnell, J.Q. and Wheeler M. (2002). "Evidence-based nutrition principles and recommendations for the treatment and prevention of diabetes and related complications (Review)", *Diabetes Care* 25: 148-198.

Gary, T.C. Ko, Hendena P.S. Wai and Joyce S.F. Tang (2006). "Effects of age on plasma glucose levels in Non-diabetic Hong Kong Chinese" *Croat. Med. J.,* 47(5): 709-713.

Ghattu, V. Krishanaveni (MBBS), J. Saperia, H.C. Jacqueline, S. Anandalhirtha L.D. Samantha, K.C. Samuel, V.R. Sargoor and D.H. Caroline (2005). "Anthropometry, glucose tolerance, and insulin concentrations in Indian children relationship to maternal glucose and insulin concentrations during pregnancy", *Diabetes Care,* 28(12)-2919-2925.

Gupta, Rajeev and Anoop Misra (2007). "Review: Type 2 diabetes in India: Regional disparities", *B.J. Diabetes Vas Dis.*, 7: 12-16.

Imkongtenla, Pongen (2017). *Risk Factors of Lifestyle Related Disease Among Ao Nagas*, unpublished thesis, University of Delhi, Delhi.

Jaroslaw, Ogonowski and Tomasz Miazgoski (2010). "Are short women at risk for gestational diabetes mellitus?" *Eur. J. Endocrinol.,* 162:491-497.

Katzmarzyk, P.T. (2008). "Physical activity data Canada", *Health Indicator,* Canada: Canada Institute of Health Information.

Klein, S., Sheard, N.F., Pi-Sunyer X., Daly A., Wylie-Rosett J., Kulkarni, K., Clark, N.G (2004). "The American Diabetes Association, the North American Association for the Study of Obesity, the American Society for Clinical Nutrition: Weight management through lifestyle modification for the prevention and management of Type 2 diabetes: rationale and strategies: a statement of the American Diabetes Association, the North American Association for the Study of Obesity, and the American Society for Clinical Nutrition", *Diabetes Care,* 27(1):2067-2073.

Lawlor, D.A., Ebrahim, S., Davey, and Smith, G. (2002). "The association between components of adult height and type 2 diabetes and insulin resistance: British women's heart and health study", *Diabetologia,* 45: 1097-1106.

Meisinger, C., Döring, A., Thorand, B., Heier, M., and Löwel, H. (2006). "Body fat distribution and risk of type 2 diabetes in the general population: are there differences between men and women? The MONICA/KORA Augsburg cohort Study." *Am. J. Clin. Nutr.*, 84 (3):483-9.

Ming Wei, M.D., MPH; Larry, W. Gibbons, M.D., M.P.H.; James B. Kampert, Ph.D.; Milton Z. Nichaman, M.D., S.D.; Steven N. Blair, P.E.D. (2000). "Low cardiorespiratory fitness and physical inactivity as predictors of mortality in men with type 2 diabetes", *Ann Intern Med,* 132(8):605-611.

Ramchandran, A., Snehalatha, C., and Viswanatham, Vijay (2002). "Burden of Type 2 diabetes and its complications—The Indian scenario", *Current Science,* 83: 1471-1476.

Sacco, R. (2013). "Accelerating progress on non-communicable disease", *Lancet,* 382 (9895): e4-e5.

Shah, Shekhar (2000). *Diabetic Made Easy*, Assam: Swapna Publishing House, Diabetes Clinic and Research Centre, and Guwahati. pp. 1-7.

Sobngwi, E., J.C.N. Mbanya, N.C. Unwin, A.P. Kengne, L. Fezeu, E.M. Minkoulou, T.J. Aspray and K.G.M.M. Alberti (2002). "Physical activity and its relationship with obesity, hypertension and diabetes in urban and rural Cameroon", *Int. J. Obes. Relat. Metab. Disord*; 26(7): 1009-16.

Sullivam, J.B.O. and Boston, M.D. (1974), "Age gradient and blood glucose level: Magnitude and clinical implication", *Diabetes*, 28(8): 713-715.

Sullivan, Patrick W., Morrato, Elaine, H., Ghushchyan, Vahram, Wyatt, Holly, R., Hill, James, O. (2005). "Obesity, inactivity, and the prevalence of diabetes and diabetes-related cardiovascular comorbidities in the U.S., 2000-2002", *Diabetes Care,* 28(7): 1599-1603.

U.S. Department of Health and Human Services (2001). *The Surgeon General's Call to Action to Prevent and Decrease Overweight and Obesity.* Rockville, MD, Public Health Service, Office of the Surgeon General.

U.S. Department of Health and Human Services (1996). Surgeon General's report on physical activity and health [article online]. Available from http://www.cdc.gov/nccdphp/sgr/sgr.htm. Accessed 15 January, 2017.

Villegas, Raquel, Xio-Ou Shu, Honglan Li, Gong Yang, Charles E. Mathews, Michael Leitzmann, Qi Li, Hui Cai, Yu-Tang Gao and Wei Zheng (2006). "Physical activity and the incidence of type 2 diabetes in the Shanghai women's health study", *Int. J. Epidemo.*, 35: 1553-1562.

Wang, Youfa, Eric B. Rimm, Meir J. Stampfer, Walter C. Willett and Frank B. Hu (2005). "Comparison of abdominal adiposity and overall obesity in predicting risk of type 2 diabetes among men", *Am. J. Clin. Nutrvol.*, 81(3):555-563.

WHO (2008). The Global Burden of Chronic Available from http://www.who.int/nutrition/topics/2_background/en/. Retrieved on: 15-03-2017, 1:40 pm.

WHO (2010). WHO classification of Obesity-Behind the Medical Headlnes. Available from http://www.thelancet.com/journals/lancet/article/PIIS0140-6736(17)32129-3/fulltext Accessed on 20th February, 2017.

WHO (2014). Global status report on non-communicable disease. Available from www.who.int/nmh/publications/ncd-status-report-2014/en/ Retrieved on: 15 03-2017, 1:37 pm.

Yadav, Vikram Singh, Shyamal Koley, Sandhu, J.S., Shishir Nigam and Puneet Arora (2007). "A study on somatotyping of patients with type 2 diabetes mellitus in Amritsar", *Anthropologist,* 9 (3): 247-249.

Part-III

Fertility and Mortality

8

Fertility and Mortality Profile among the Khasi of Meghalaya

Duka Devi Chhetri

Introduction

Demography is the scientific study of human populations, primarily with respect to their size, structure, and current and future development. It also deals with the study of population quality. Absolute number of persons (or the size of the population), age, sex, demographic events like births, deaths, marriages, divorce, migration etc. are important demographic factors. In demographic trend, fertility and morality are important features for calculating population movement. Fertility is known to vary rather widely among the adults of every population. Such fertility variation between different groups is called differential fertility. Mortality variation between different groups is called differential mortality. The numbers of births and deaths that take place are themselves influenced by the size and age distribution of the population. The difference between the number of births and deaths, natural change, is a key determinant of population size and growth. If there are more births than deaths, a population will experience natural increase. Conversely, if more deaths occur than births, a population will experience natural decrease (Reddy and Sudha, 2010). Historically, the process of gradual change from a situation of relatively high fertility and high mortality to one of relatively low fertility and low mortality, observed in many countries, is called demographic transition.

The demographic transition theory (DTT) was arguably the founding paradigm of international demography. The demographic transition theory suggested that the fertility transition would result from structural changes linked to a general modernization process that included economic development, industrialization, and urbanization (Heuveline, 2003). Apart from death rate and birth rate, migration is also an important factor for the change in demographic structure of a population. During the time of hunter and gatherer, human population is very small and it remained integrated well within the boundaries of the ecosystem/landscape. With settlements appearing with the advent of agriculture about 10,000 years ago, the exploitative phase of the human population started growing rapidly.

The world experienced dramatic population growth during the twentieth century, with the number of inhabitants doubling from 3 to 6 billion between 1960 and 2000. India, too, saw a very rapid population growth during this period from 448 million to 1.04 billion and to 1.21 billion in 2010. The effects of past and projected future demographic change on economic growth in India are the main focus. Global population grew at roughly 2 per cent per annum from 1960-2000, a level that is unsustainable in the long term, as it translates into population doubling every 35 years. India's population is currently growing at a rate of 1.4 per cent per year, far surpassing China's rate of 0.7 per cent. The differential between India and China will result in India surpassing China with respect to population size in less than 20 years (Bloom, 2011). While most of the developing countries perceive their fertility as too high, while many developed countries are concerned for too low fertility rates (Hartmann, 2010).

Fertility and mortality are fundamental determinants of population growth in order to understand the changes in human population structure. Studies all over the world have brought forth evidences in support of contention that the socio-economic and socio-cultural milieus of a population have tremendous impact on the fertility and mortality component of that population (Kapoor *et al.,* 2003). Biological as well as Socio-cultural factors are responsible for differential.

Only few studies have been carried out concerning this research area of anthropological interest in this part of country. Therefore, we have undertaken a study on differential fertility and mortality among Khasi population of the Saiden village, Re-Bhoi district of Meghalaya. Fertility and mortality rate in the study population was conducted in relation to socio-economic factors such as family planning, marital status, economic condition, occupation, education level of the women.

Materials and Methods

Period and Duration of the Fieldwork

The present fieldwork study was conducted in Saiden village, Re-Bhoi district of Meghalaya from 20th January to 8th February, 2015. No statistical sampling technique was applied in the selection of individual and household for the present study. I manage to collect data from 71 women by survey of house to house visit. Table below shows the brief census of the village based on the data gather during the course of fieldwork. The traditional Anthropological ethnographic method of participant observation was the main strategy in collecting the data. Both the daily life of Khasi and special rituals, festival was conducted along with many formal and informal interviews with villagers.

Nature of demographic data collected was based on the parameters suggested by the World Health Organisation (1964-1968). These are as follows:

Individual records: It includes name of the informants, its relationship with the head of the household, tribes, religion, total numbers of family members, age, sex, marital status, place of birth and place of residence etc.

Fertility: Data on fertility includes the pregnancy history of each woman, present age of mothers, age at marriage, age at first child birth, total number of conception, total number of live births, birth order, sex and marital status of each offspring.

Mortality: Data on mortality includes number of dead children, sex, age at death, causes of death, number of reproductive wastage (still birth, spontaneous and induce abortion) etc. In the present study, we have divided morality into two groups, namely infant mortality and juvenile mortality.

Income groups: Data on household income were collected directly from the head of the household or the women who interviewed. They were cross-checked taking into considerations some aspects of socio-economic conditions like housing condition, type of occupation, land holding. Per capita income of household was classified into following three categories:

- Above 75th percentile (>Rs. 5674) = High income group (HIG)
- Between 75th-50th percentile (Rs. 2500–5674) = Middle income group (MIG)
- Below 50th percentile (<Rs. 2500) = Lower income group (LIG)

Educational level: Data on educational attainment of individuals were classified into four categories, namely primary, secondary, higher secondary and graduate and above. The primary level of education includes those individuals who studied up to class V. In the secondary level of education, we included those individuals who attended standard VI to X. Higher secondary level of education included those who attended standard XI to XII. In the graduate and above level of education, we included those individuals who have completed graduation and those pursuing higher studies.

Method of Data Collection

The entire demographic data were collected from 71 women through interview using structural schedules visiting house to house survey. Information on age, sex, marital status, occupation, place of birth, place of residence etc., was collected. The fertility and mortality schedules was completed by filing information on the numbers of conception, numbers of live births, birth orders, age, sex, marital status of each offspring, numbers of death children, cause of death, if any, reproductive wastage (abortion and still births) through in-depth interview with each of the married women. Special attention also made to collect data on socio-economic parameters, like occupation, household income, household expenditure, educational attainment of household members especially married women, religious affiliation, age at marriage, awareness and adoption of the family planning method etc.

Statistical Analysis

All the parameters taken were analysed statistically to find out the mean and the standard error. In order to test the level of significance, *t*-test, ANOVA and Chi-square test have been used. MS-Excel software was used for all statistical analyses of the present research.

Results

The findings of the present study are discussed below:

Table 8.1 shows the completed family size among the Khasi females of the present study. For the measuring completed family size, we have considered only those women who were aged 40 years and above. The Table shows that the mean number of live births and surviving children to such mothers were 3.11± 0.19 and 2.44±0.20 respectively.

Table 8.1: Live Birth by Age Group of Married Females of the Saiden Village

Number of women above 40 years	*Number of live births of children*	*Number of surviving children*	*Mean live birth of children ±SE*	*Mean surviving children ±SE*
32	119	89	3.11±0.19	2.44±0.20

Source: Author's Study.

Table 8.2 shows the mean number of live births per mother. Table indicates that the mean number of live births per mother in the study population was more or less the same in all the age groups, with slightly higher in the age group =24 (3.38±1.27). The mean number of live birth 3.07±0.59, 3.21±0.15, 3.13±0.09, 3.11±0.08 and 3.14±0.03 were found in the age groups 25-29 years, 30-34 years, 35-39 years, 40-44 years, 45+years respectively.

Table 8.2: Number of Live Births by Age at Marriage of the Females of Saiden Village.

Age of marriage	*No. of mothers*	*No. of live births*	*Mean live birth ±SE*
≤19	–	–	–
20-24	3	4	1.33± 1.27
>25	68	217	3.19± 0.14

$t = 3.023$; $df = 2$; $p < 0.05$

Source: Author's Study.

The mean number of live births by age at marriage of females is given in Table 8.5. It was found that the mean number of live births was lower among females who married at the age between 20-24 years (1.33±1.27) than those who married above 25 years of age (3.19±0.14).

Table 8.3: Infant Mortality, Juvenile Mortality and Reproductive Wastage

Parameters	*Frequency*
Number of mothers	71
Total number of pregnancies	258
Number of live births	221
Number of deaths before 1 year	5
Number of deaths between1 to 14 years	2
Infant mortality rate %	2.26
Juvenile mortality rate%	0.09
Total number of reproductive wastage	19
Reproductive wastage %	7.36

Source: Author's Study.

Table 8.3 shows the frequency of infant mortality, juvenile mortality and reproductive wastage of the study population. Out of 221 live births of the mother of all ages, five live births died before the age of 1 year and two live births died between 1 to 14 years of age. The frequency of the infant and juvenile mortality rate was 2.26 per cent and 0.09 per cent respectively. It indicates that mortality rate especially infant mortality is little high than juvenile mortality in this population. The table further indicates that the rate of reproductive wastage out of total pregnancies was 7.36 per cent.

Table 8.4: Age Specific Fertility Rate among Females of Saiden Village

Age group of mothers	*Number of mothers*	*Number of live births*	*Age specific rate*
15–19	–	–	–
20–24	71	221	3.10
25–29	68	217	3.19
30–34	63	210	3.33
35–39	52	184	3.53
40–45	40	148	3.70
45+	26	103	3.96
Total fertility rate (TFR)			**20.81**

Source: Author's Study.

Table 8.4 illustrated the age specific fertility rate of the married females of the population. The Table shows that the age specific fertility rate was more or less the same in all the age groups, but slightly higher value was found among mothers above 45+ years of age (3.96). The age fertility rates 3.10, 3.19, 3.33, 3.53 and 3.70 were found among females aged between 20–24 years, 25–29 years, 30–34 years, 35–39 years and 40–45 years respectively. The total fertility rate (TFR), that is the sum of total of age specific fertility rate was 20.81.

Table 8.5: Fertility Rate by Educational Level of the Mother of the Saiden Village

Education	*No. of mothers*	*No. of live births*	*No. of surviving*	*Mean live births ±SE*	*Mean surviving ±SE*
Primary	31	121	87	3.90±0.20	2.71±0.22
Secondary	26	73	65	2.80±0.25	2.50± 0.25
Graduate+	14	27	22	1.92±0.40	1.57±0.40

F = 5.071; df = 2; p<0.05 (live births) F = 1.383; df = 2, p<0.05
Source: Author's Study.

The mean number of live births and surviving children according to educational level of the mothers are mention in Table 8.5. The mean number of live births 3.90±0.20 was found higher among the females who attained primary education. This was followed by mean number of live births 2.80±0.25 and 1.92±0.40 among the secondary and graduate and above level of education respectively. The Table further indicates that mean number of surviving children 2.71±0.22 and 2.50±0.25 were more or less the same between the primary level of education and secondary level of education. The mean surviving children 1.57±0.40 was found among the females who attained the graduate and above level of education. It is clearly seen from Table 8.5 that the mean number of live births and surviving children tends to decrease with the increasing educational level among others.

Table 8.6: Fertility Rate by the Income Level of the Family of Saiden Village

Income	*No. of mothers*	*No. of live births*	*No. of surviving*	*Mean live birth± SE*	*Mean surviving±SE*
Low	33	127	91	3.84±0.19	2.75± 0.21
Middle	20	62	55	3.10± 0.27	2.75± 0.27
High	18	32	28	1.78±0.37	1.55 ±0.35

F = 6.067; p<0.05 (live birth) F = 2.073; p>0.05(surviving birth)
Source: Author's Study.

Table 8.6 shows the mean live birth and surviving children by the income level of the households. The mean live birth 3.84±0.19 was found slightly higher in low income family followed by middle income family (3.1±0.27) and high income family (1.78±0.37). The differences in the mean live births in different income levels were statistically significant ($F = 6.067$; $p<0.05$). However, the higher frequency of mean surviving children was found the same in both the low income family (2.75±0.21) and middle income family (2.75±0.27). The lowest frequency of mean surviving children (1.55±0.35) was found among the females belonging to the higher income family.

Table 8.7: Infant Mortality Rate by Income Level of the Family of the Saiden Village

Income	*No. of live births*	*No. of infants*	*Infant mortality*
Low income	127	3	2.36%
Middle income	62	2	3.23%
High income	32	–	–

$\chi^2 = 0.114$; df = 1; $p>0.05$
Source: Author's Study.

Table 8.7 shows the infant mortality rate by the level of income of the family. The frequency of infant mortality rate was slightly higher among the middle income family (3.23%) than low income group (2.36%).

Table 8.8: Infant Mortality Rate by Educational Level of Mothers of the Saiden Village

Education	*Number of live births*	*Number of infant deaths*	*Infant morality %*
Primary	121	3	2.48%
Secondary	73	2	2.73%
Graduate+	27	–	–

$\chi^2 = 0.011$; df = 1; $p>0.05$
Source: Author's Study.

The infant mortality rate in relation to educational level of the mother of the present study is given in Table 8.8. Table 8.8 shows that the infant mortality rate was more or less the same between the primary (2.48%) and secondary (2.73%) level of education of the mothers. The differences in infant mortality in different educational levels were not statistically significant ($\chi^2 = 0.011$; df = 1; $p>0.05$).

Discussion and Conclusion

The mean age at marriage and mean age at first child birth in the present study is found to be significantly lower in females than males. The number of live births is higher than the mean number of surviving children among women who have completed family size, i.e. mothers who married only once and live continuously in wedlock till attainment of the age 40 years. The present study shows that the mean numbers of live birth per mothers of all the age groups are found more or less the same. Similarly, the mean numbers of surviving children per mother of all the age groups are also found more the or less the same. The mean number of live birth is higher among women married at age of twenty five years and above. The infant mortality rate is higher than the juvenile mortality rate. The frequency of the reproductive wastage in the present study population is lower than that other study (Haloi, 2014). The fertility rate in the present population is moderately high. The probable reason could be due to the reproductive behaviour and reproductive decision, inadequate facilities of family planning in the village, lack of proper education about family planning method etc. (Saikia, 2005).

Demographic parameters such as fertility and mortality are reported to have associated with various biological and socio-economic factors. Socio-economic status of the family plays an important role in fertility and mortality rate of the population. The present study shows that fertility rate is higher among women belong to the low income family. It further indicates that the fertility rate tends to decrease with increasing the level of the income of the family. Similarly, the number of surviving children also decreases with increasing the level of income of the family. Several studies suggested that the economic conditions influence the fertility rate of an individual (Dey and Goswami, 2009). A better educated woman not withstanding her residence may experience different fertility to uneducated woman (Ushie *et al.*, 2011). Educated women are aware and more knowledgeable about the desired family size, family planning, planned numbers of births etc. Educated and employed women are more likely to use contraception than those who have little education and who are not employed (Al-kandari, 2007). Further, educated women are likely to be less dependent on their sons as sources of social status and old age security and this too may lead to the reduction in family size.

Infant mortality is slightly higher in the middle income group than the lower income group. There is no case of infant mortality in the higher income group in the present research. The mortality rate shows more or less the same between the primary level of education and secondary level of education of the mothers. The present study further indicated that there is no case of infant mortality among the higher educated women. Educated women are likely to be more knowledgeable about nutrition, hygienic and health of the children (Marthi *et al.,* 1995). The relation between female educations with fertility has a crucial bearing change in the fertility and mortality rate. Indeed, female education plays a key role in the social development approach (Dreze, 2001). However, education does not play an important role in infant mortality rate in the present research.

The people of Saiden village has always connect health with cultural beliefs. They believed that medicines along with prayers would help in curing any disease. The residents of the village were believers of black magic that could even take some one's life. The health according to them was due to black magic. The villagers were very much aware of the healthy way of living; the village was awarded the cleanest villages in the Re-Bhoi district of Meghalaya.

In conclusion, the present study among Khasi women of Saiden village highlights the fertility and mortality rates in relation with certain socio-economic conditions. The mean number of live births and surviving children in all the age groups are found more or less the same. However, the number of live births is higher than the mean number of surviving children among women who have completed family size. Family income plays an important role in determining the fertility and mortality rate. However, the education level of them others does not indicate much influenced on the fertility and mortality rate in the present research.

Acknowledgements

I will like to extend my sincere thanks to all the women of Saiden Village of Meghalaya. For their time, patient and cooperation.

References

Al Kandari, Y.Y. (2007). "Fertility and its relationship with socio-cultural factor in Kuwaiti society", *Eastern Mediterranean Health Journal*, 13(6):1364-1371.

Angeles, L. (2010). "Demographic transitions: analysing the effect of mortality and fertility", *Journal of Population Ecology*, 23:99-120.

Bharathi, K. (2014). "Impact of consanguinity on fertility and mortality", *Journal of Humanities and Social Science*, 19(4):39-42.

Bloom, D.E. (2011). *Population dynamic in India and Implication for Economic Growth.* Working paper series 65, Harvard School of Public Health.

Breierova, L. adn Duflo, E. (2002). The impact of education on fertility and child mortality: Do father really matter less than mother? Available from http://economics.mit.edu/files/738. (Accessed on 15 May, 2015).

Census (2011). *Meghalaya Profile,* Available from http://www.census2011.co.in/census/state/meghalaya.html (Accessed on 15 May, 2015).

Chaudhari, S. (2012). "The desire for sons and excess fertility: A household-level analysis of parity progression in India", *International Perspectives on Sexual and Reproductive Health*, 38(4):178-185.

Dey, S. and Goswami, S. (2009). "Fertility pattern and its correlates in North East India", *Journal of Human Ecology*, 26(2):145-152.

Dikshit, R., Dikshit, K. and Jutta, K. (2014). *North East India: Land, People and Economy*, New York: Springer.

Dreze, J. (2001). "Fertility, education development: evidence from India", *Population and Development Review*, 27(1):33-63.

Haloi, A. (2014). "Fertility differentials of marriage and their reproductive wastage in a Muslim population of rural northeast India", *Human Biology Review*, 3(1):1-14.

Hartmann, A.M. (2010). *Fertility and Economic Growth,* Available from http://pure.au.dk/portal-asb-student/files/12445/Thesis_AM-Hartmann.pdf (Accessed on 20 May, 2015).

Heuveline, P. (2003). *Mortality and Fertility Interactions: New Insights from Recent Population Dynamics in Cambodia,* Available from http://www.prgs.edu/content/dam/rand/www/external/labour/seminars/adp/pdfs/adpheuveline.pdf (Accessed on 15 May, 2015).

Jones, G. (2012). "Late marriage and low fertility in Singapore: The limits of policy", *The Japanese Journal of Population*, 10(1):89-101.

Kapoor, A.K., Kshatriya, G.K., and Kopoor, S. (2003). "Fertility and mortality differential among the population group of Himalayas", *Human Biology*, 75 (5):729-747.

Karaman, D.D., and Goldstein, J.R. (2010). The increasing importance of economic conditions on fertility, MPIDR working papers WP-2010-014, Max Plank, Institute for Demographic Research, Rostock, Germany.

Karki, Y.B., and Krishna, R. (2008). *Factors Responsible for the Rapid Decline of Fertility in Nepal—An Interpretation*, Available from http://un.org.np/data-coll/Health–Publications/200NDHSFertility decline.pdf (Accessed on 20 May, 2015).

Kayastha, S.L. (2007). *Geography of Population*, New Delhi: Rawat Publication.

Kenya National Bureau of Statistics, (2015). *Demographic and Health Survey*, Available from http://dhsprogram.com/pubs/pdf/PR55/PR55.pdf (Accessed on 20 May, 2015).

Kullar, D.R. (2012). *India: A Comprehensive Geography*, New Delhi: Kalyani Publishers.

9

Infant Mortality

An Anthropological Analysis among Tribal of Krushnanagar in Khordha District, Odisha

Sanghamitra Sethi

Introduction

Anthropological studies on health of tribal give rich ethnographic details about their cultural practices, perception and behavioural aspects. The World Health Organization (WHO) states that the enjoyment of the highest attainable standard of health is one of the fundamental rights of every human being without distinction of races, religion, political belief, economic or social conditions. Health is multi-dimensional approach. The WHO envisages three specific dimensions, the physical, mental and social. The state of physical health implies the notion of perfect functioning of body. Mental health is not mere absence of mental illness. Good mental health is the ability to respond to the many varied experiences of life with flexibility and a sense of purpose. Social well-being implies harmony and integration within the individual between each individual and other members of society and between individual and the world in which they live. Health is basic requirement not only for the fulfilment of human aspiration, but also for the enjoyment of all mankind of better quality of life. It is also indispensable for balanced development of the individual within the family and as a part of the community and the nation. Health of women is a prerequisite for development and is one of the important indicators of their status. The accessibility, affordability and availability of health services are needed to understand the health of the tribal populations, especially maternal and child health. Deaths of infant are mostly in account of the poor health status of the mother during pre-natal and post-natal period and also lack of proper experience in rearing infant (Kalla & Joshi, 2004).

In order to develop realistic health plans based on the felt needs of tribal women and children. Infant health shapes child health which in turn powerfully influences adult health. The Department of Health has identified five key actions for the successful delivery of the infant mortality target. The contributions of biological and socio-environmental factors to the cause of morbidity or mortality are not easy to measure. Rural population that have satisfactory sanitation, water supply and medical facilities, are known to have death rates that are lower than those in urban areas (Karkal, 1985). One of these actions is to "develop a plan to strengthen the evidence base about interventions to reduce infant mortality." The infant mortality rate is defined as the total number of infant deaths per 1,000 live births in a specified period of time. Infant deaths are divided into two groups: those that occurring at less than 28 days after birth are referred as neonatal deaths; and those occurring after 28 days and over, but within one year is referred as post-neonatal deaths. Infant mortality rates have for a long time been used as country or regional level proxy indicators of socio-economic position. Infant mortality has also long been regarded as an important indicator of population health. Neonatal mortality rates are especially sensitive to events during pregnancy, delivery and in the neonatal period care given to mothers and their babies. Post-neonatal mortality is thought to be influenced to a greater extent by parental circumstances, including their socio-economic position, and the care they provide for their infant. Higher neo-natal mortality is leading to high per cent of IMR and still birth. High child mortality rates in the tribal areas and urban slums (Bang, Reddy & Deshmukh, 2002). First birth order carries high risk of infant death due to early age at marriage, teenage pregnancy. The risk of death was higher for infants born within the birth intervals of less than two years compared with those born beyond spacing of two or more years (Patel, Kumar, Godara, Desai, 2013).

Child mortality rate decreases with increase in mother's education (Das & Das, 2015). Female literacy rate have a positive impact in reducing infant mortality rate (Shetty & Shetty, 2014). Low age at marriage along with low age at first delivery (18-20 years) indicates the long reproductive period before maturity, which may be associated with infant mortality, benign and harmful traditional birth-related practices of having delivery at home, attended by untrained personnel, cutting the umbilical cord by unhygienic instruments, treatment of umbilical stump by oil, discarding the colostrum and breastfeeding their infants, regularly after initial delays, increases the risk of dying of the newborns (Verma, Saha, Kumar, 2005). No knowledge of identifying sick neonatal symptoms is the main cause of infant death. Among the neonatal deaths, women still preferred delivery at home compared to hospital. Practice of essential newborn care was not observed among neonatal deaths, either home or hospital delivered. Among neonatal deaths delivered at home, this non-practice of essential newborn practice was more common. There are high prevalence of home deliveries and inaccessibility of neonatal care in tribal area (Garikipati, Babu, Pant, Murthy, 2013).

Reproductive and Child Health (RCH) programme is a wide flagship programme under the umbrella of the Government of India's (GoI) National Health Mission (NHM) to deliver the RCH targets for reduction of maternal and infant mortality and total fertility rates. RCH programme aims to reduce social and geographical disparities in access to and utilization of quality reproductive, maternal, newborn, child and adolescent health services. Launched in April 2005 in partnership with the State Governments, RCH is consistent with Government of India's National Population Policy-2000, the National Health Policy-2001 and the Millennium Development Goals. Six key components of the RCH programmes are: Maternal Health, Child Health, Nutrition, Family Planning, Adolescent Health (AH) and PCPNDT. In order to address newborn health in high priority districts Newborn Care Corners (NBCCs) are being established at delivery points to provide essential newborn care at birth, while Special Newborn Care Units (SNCUs) and Newborn Stabilization Units (NBSUs) provide care for sick newborns in these poorest priority districts with respect to health indicators. Complete elimination of out of pocket expenses with provision of free transport, drugs, diagnostics and diet to all sick newborns and infants is being ensured in the country through Janani-Shishu Suraksha Karyakrama (JSSK).

Table 9.1: List of Beneficiary JSSK

Sl. No.	*Years*	*JSSK*	*Institutional delivery*	*Home delivery*	*Family Planning*
1.	2015	10	11	5	5
2.	2016	5	10	2	7

Source: Present Fieldwork, Krushnanagar.

Study Area and People

According to the 2011 Census, Khordha district has a population of 2,251,673 of which male and female were 1,167,137 and 1,084,536 respectively. The village Krushnanagar is located under Daruthenga Gram Panchayat under Chandaka Police Station in Bhubaneswar block of Khordha district. The Sabar people are one of the Scheduled Tribes in India. They are mainly found in Odisha, Jharkhand, Chhattisgarh, Madhya Pradesh and West Bengal.

Materials and Methods

Anthropological studies are characterized by their holistic approach of study based on first-hand information collected through fieldwork. The chapter is based on the field study among Sabar in Khordha District, Odisha. Purposive sampling technique is used to collect data from the respondent. The women having children, pregnant women, mother-in-laws were interviewed. The anganwadi worker and ASHA also interviewed to get the changing picture about delivery. The study emphasis on Infant Mortality: An Anthropological Analysis among Tribals of Krushnanagar in Khordha district, Odisha. This chapter aims at a critical analysis of the trends in infant mortality and associated different causes of infant death. This chapter is a qualitative study based on primary data collected through Interview Scheduled, In-depth interview, Case Study and Focus Group Discussions (FGDs). Secondary information has collected from various documents such as books, magazines, journals and old research papers as well as from internet etc. The study covered 95 households and the population is about 599 out of which male (240) and female (359) out of total population under-five children (57) and infant (11).

Results

The tribal people of India in general and Odisha in particular basically

Table 9.2: List of Pregnancy, Delivery and Infant Death

Sl. No.	Category	Years				
		2012	2013	2014	2015	2016
1.	Pregnancy	3	13	19	18	11
2.	Delivery	9	11	6	16	12
3.	Infant Death	–	1	–	3	–

Source: Present Fieldwork, Krushnanagar

Table 9.3: Child Delivery Status in Odisha,

Sl. No.	Type of Delivery	Total	Male	Female
1.	Institutional	572799	296021	276778
2.	Trained Personnel	101346	56295	45051
3.	Untrained Personnel	28701	15620	13081
4.	Others	64214	33545	30669
5.	**Total**	**767060**	**401481**	**36557**

Source: Directorate of Health and Family Welfare.

lived in the natural surrounding within the hill, forest and river side. They have accustomed with the environment and plant species from which extract their livelihood and day-to-day needs and basic necessity of life. Though the tribals of Krushnanagar are migrated from Mayurbhanj, Cuttack and Keonjhar district but still they reside close to the Chandaka forest. So, they prefer different Ayurveda medicines for curing the diseases. But now due to the impact of education and awareness campaign by health worker the people prefer to acquire modern health care services. The rate of infant mortality in the case of home delivery by traditional birth attendant/*dhai* is high because use of instrument by *dhai* may cause septic as she cut the umbilical cord with the help of blade or knife. But, after immunization programme and cash assistance programme of government and awareness created by health worker motivate people to prefer institutional delivery.

Five Year Plans Focusing on Child Development

In the First Five Year Plan (1951-56) importance is given to social welfare. The Focus imposed on welfare of children and also of physically and mentally disabled. In the Second Five Year Plan 2100 Maternity and Child Health Centres were set up to provide primary health services. In Fourth Five Year Plan (1969-74) measures taken to control and eradicate communicable diseases, to provide curative and preventive health services in rural areas through the establishment of a Primary Health Centre in each community development block. In Fifth Five Year Plan (1974-78) ICDS was launched with a six package services, like health check-up, immunization, referral services, supplementary feeding, non-formal pre-school education and health and nutrition education for children below 6 years and expectant and nursing mothers through Anganwadi centre. In Sixth Five Year Plan (1980-85) the National Health Policy was adopted to improve health care and reduce infant mortality and child mortality and priority to immunization etc. In Seventh Five Year Plan (1985-90) most extensive programme was undertaken for maternal and child care, importance given on sanitation and hygiene, family planning etc. Immunization programme adopted to cope with six lethal diseases, viz. diphtheria, whooping cough, tetanus, polio, measles and childhood tuberculosis. In Eighth Five Year Plan (1992-97) plan and programme are formulated for development, protection of child, NPA formulated focusing on children and girl child specially abolish of gender bias. Priority was given to reduce high infant and under five mortality and morbidity. The Ninth Five Year Plan (1997-2002) measures taken for promoting the overall development of the young children, especially the Girl child and the mothers all over the country; arresting the declining sex-ratio and curb its related problems of female foeticide and female infanticide, reduce Infant mortality rate. The Tenth Five Year Plan had objectives to reduce the mortality, fertility and rate of population growth. The target was to reduce the number of infant mortality rate (IMR) 45/1000 live birth by 2007 and the rate still reduce to 28/1000 live birth by 2012. The reduction of IMR to 2/1000 live birth by 2007 and reach to 1/1000 live birth by 2012. In the Eleventh Five Year Plan (2007-12) for reducing infant mortality, focus was on Home Based Newborn Care (HBNC) complemented by Integrated Management of Neonatal and Childhood Illnesses. HBNC was provided by a trained Community Health Worker (such as ASHA) who guide and support the mother, family and TBA in the care of the newborn, and attend to the newborn at home if she is sick.

The major objectives of Twelfth Five Year Plan was the reduction of IMR to 25. India was targeting to have an IMR of 36 by 35 and 32 by 2017. To achieve the goal various majors, such, as training provided to skilled birth attendant, traditional birth attendant must be trained, monitor the quality of institutional deliveries and breast feeding was encouraged.

The Government of India has taken initiatives to reduce infant mortality rate of India. But, still the goal is not achieved. The rate is still high.

Table 9.4: Infant Mortality Rate (PER-1000) in India and Odisha

Sl. No.	*Year*	*Total*		*Male*		*Female*	
		India	*Odisha*	*India*	*Odisha*	*India*	*Odisha*
1.	2008	53	69	52	68	55	70
2.	2009	50	65	49	65	52	66
3.	2010	47	61	46	60	49	61
4.	2011	44	57	43	55	46	58
5.	2012	42	53	41	52	44	54
6.	2013	40	51	39	50	42	52

Source: SRS Statistics Report 2013.

Causes of Infant Mortality in Krushnanagar

From the field study it is found that there are number of causes behind the infant death. These are the followings causes:

Social Factors

- ***Education***: Children born to mothers with at least few years of schooling have more chances to survive. IMR among children born to illiterate mothers have been consistently higher than those born to educated mothers. However, the association between maternal education and child mortality becomes significant only when maternal education exceeds 8 years of schooling.
- ***Safe drinking water***: The children living in families who accessed drinking water from a safe source as compared to those who accessed drinking water from an unsafe source. The children suffered from infectious disease.
- ***Use of toilet***: Access to an improved toilet is potentially an important determinant of infant and child mortality.
- ***Clean cooking fuel***: The type of cooking fuel used in a household could affect mortality, if children spend a great deal of time where cooking takes place, the use of cooking fuel that emits harmful smoke could elevate their risk of respiratory disease and hence mortality. Secondly, children

born to mothers who have exposure to smoke during pregnancy are more likely to be low birth weight and therefore, at a higher risk of death.

- ***Traditional believe system*:** The tribal have their own culture and belief system. They put a number of restrictions on pregnant women regarding the life style and food pattern. They restricted to take non-vegetarian food to the pregnant women and also prefer to give birth by traditional birth attendant. And even they do not give attention to the immunization provided for the children during the new-natal and post neo-natal period.
- ***Age*:** Children born to adolescent mothers are at higher risk. Infant mortality rates are highest among mothers under 20 years of age. The rates are lowest among the children born to mothers between the ages of 20-24, remain reduce to 25-34 years of age and the rate is increased after 35.
- ***Spacing between births*:** Children born less than two years after the first delivery are less likely to survive. There is a consistent and significant impact of birth intervals less than 24 months on child survival. A child born within 24 months of the previous child has higher risk of dying within the neonatal period and in the post-neonatal period. The risk further increases sharply if the previous child has died. A short birth interval not only increases mortality risk of the subsequently born children, but also of those born earlier.
- ***Maternal nutrition status*:** Nutritional status of mother has a direct impact on infant mortality.
- ***Birth weight*:** It is an important indicator of a child's vulnerability to the risk of childhood illness and chances of survival. In the absence of birth weight, a mother's subjective assessment of the size of the baby at birth is a useful proxy for birth weight. Children whose birth weight is less than 2.5 kilograms or children reported to be 'very small' or 'smaller than average' are considered to have a higher than average risk of early childhood death.
- ***Attendance at childbirth*:** Deliveries attended by health professionals have a lower risk. The neonatal mortality is lowest for children delivered at home by health professionals and was highest for children delivered at home by traditional birth attendants. Mortality among those delivered in a hospital is very less.

- ***Economic factor***: The persons those who are living below poverty line may found the high risk of infant mortality. As they are not able to provide nutritious and healthy diet to their children. Due to insufficient economy parents are not live in a well condition house pattern, safe drinking water and sanitation facilities which in terms the children suffered from different communicable and non-communicable diseases. In the present study the couple have belongs to BPL category.

Role of Health Worker: One of the key components of the National Rural Health Mission is to provide every village in the country with a trained female community health activist.

- ***ASHA***: India's poor marginalized tribal people have far worse health indicators than the general population. Most tribal people live in remote rural hamlets in hilly, forested or desert areas where illiteracy, physical environment, malnutrition, inadequate access to potable water, and lack of personal hygiene and sanitation make them more vulnerable to disease. One of the key components of the National Health Mission is to provide every village in the country with a trained female community health activist (ASHA). ASHA provides information related to the health issues and on existing health services to the community. ASHA motivating the women to give birth in public hospital, encouraging family planning, maintaining demographic records, transferring and accompanying with the pregnant women to the hospital, improving village sanitation. The role of ASHA regulated towards the improving the health of mother and reduce the mortality rate of both mother and infant.
- ***Auxiliary Nurse Midwives (ANM)***: ANM is a village level female health worker who is a first contact person between the community and the health services. ANM regarded as the grassroots workers in the health pyramid. ANM provides primary health care to the community. Holding weekly/ fortnightly meeting with ASHA to discuss the activities undertaken during the week/fortnight. Acting as a resource person along with Anganwadi Worker (AWW) for the training of ASHA. Participating and guiding in organising Health Days at Anganwadi Centre. Utilising ASHA in motivating the

pregnant women for coming to Sub-Centre for initial check-ups. ASHA helps ANMs in bringing married couples to Sub-Centres for adopting family planning. Guiding ASHA in motivating pregnant women for taking full course of iron folic acid (IFA) tablets and TT injections, etc. In tribal where transport facility is poor ANM conduct delivery.

- ***Anganwadi worker*:** The Ministry of Women and Child Development has laid down guidelines for the responsibilities of Anganwadi workers (AWW). Anganwadi workers are extremely important, like providing health and nutrition education to the families, motivating couple for family planning and she take care of newborn babies and ensure that all children below the age of 6 are immunized. She is providing antenatal care for pregnant women and ensuring that they are immunized against tetanus.

Findings

The study was undertaken in Krushnanagar, a tribal village in Khordha district. From the study it found that due to the health worker motivation couples show interest in family planning. In 2015, 5 couples and in 2016, 7 couples respectively adopt family planning. A major population prefer to give birth in the public hospital. From the above discussion it was observed that health is a part of culture in primitive society. Health is incorporated with social, psychological and cultural aspect. It incorporated with the traditional knowledge which comes from the culture of a definite society. In primitive society the social life, knowledge, practices and health lies in a single line. Each culture has its own characteristics perception of disease and thus its unique hygienic mask. The people obey some restriction on the foods during and after pregnancy which cause malnutrition among infant. The women still delivery at home by traditional birth attendant. The health workers also aware them regarding health issues, sanitation and hygiene and different scheme of government for maternal and child which promote them to lead a healthy life.

Conclusion

The infant mortality rate in Krushnanagar has changed. Several decade ago the tribal are practice their indigenous knowledge regarding the health issues. They preferred traditional birth attendant and different Ayurvedic medicine. But, now the people perception regarding health and modern medical facilities, but the percentage was not a catchy one. They prefer Institutional deliveries and took medicine and also nutrition food during and after pregnancy. Under the project ICDS and MAMATA scheme the pregnant and lactose mother get financial assistance and nutritious food. They are conscious about the health and their children. They prefer to go hospital at the time of illness. The mother took the medicine; vaccine and immunization also give the children till the age of five.

Acknowledgements

A part of this paper has been presented at the National seminar on "Role of Anthropology in Public Health", at Habra, West Bengal held on March 18-19, 2017. The author acknowledges the support of Department of Anthropology, Utkal University, Odisha and special thanks to village informant, Health worker, Anganwadi worker.

References

Bang, Abhay, M.H. Reddy and M.D. Deshmukh (2002). "Child mortality in Maharashtra", *Economic and Political Weekly*, Vol. 37, No. 49 (December 7-13, 2002).

Das, N., and Das, R. (2015). "A study on cause of death among the tribal children of Udalguri district, Assam", *International Journal of Medical Science and Public Health*, *4*(8): 1060-1065

Garikipati, U., Babu, G.R., Pant, H., and Murthy, G. (2013). "A study of infant deaths in tribal area of Andhra Pradesh, India", *Global Journal of Medicine and Public Health,* Vol. 2, Issue 4.

Kalla, A.K. and Joshi, P.C. (2004). *Tribal Health and Medicines,* New Delhi: Concept Publishing Company Pvt. Ltd.

Karkal, M. (1985). "Maternal and infant mortality", *Economic and Political Weekly*, Vol. 20, No. 43 (October 26, 1985).

Patel, A., P. Kumar, N. Godara and V.K. Desai (2013). "Infant Death-data disparity and use of ante, intra and post-natal services utilization: An experience from tribal areas of Gujarat", *Indian Journal of Community Medicine*, 38(3): 152-156.

Shetty, A., and Shetty, S. (2014). "The impact of female literacy on infant mortality rate in Indian States". *Current Pediatric Research*, 18(1), 49-56.

Verma, A., K.B. Saha and D. Kumar (2005). "Infant mortality in tribals of central India," *Current Science*, 89(4).

10

Differential Fertility and Mortality among the Vadabalija Women of Annavaram Village in Visakhapatnam District, Andhra Pradesh

Mong Fing Lepcha

Introduction

Population to a demographer refers to an aggregate number of people possessing some specified characteristics within a precisely defined area. Fertility and mortality are termed as the fundamental determinants of demography. There are various factors that have deeper impact on fertility and mortality, socio-economic and socio-cultural being the important ones on the list (Kapoor *et al.*, 2003). Apart from the duo biological factors also has an important role in fertility and mortality rates (Reddy and Sudha, 2010). Study also shows that the changes in birth rate and death rate are correlated with modernization (Heuveline, 2003). Few other scholars tried to relate the change in birth rate and death rate with the cultural practices that encouraged high birth rate, but along with the modernization the concern for better health started to be a reality (Notestein, 1945). Marriage rate, age at marriage, marriage pattern and widowhood are also considered as important factors regulating fertility. Marriage rates are declining with modernization where fast pace of life and increasing complexities in entire socio-economic endeavour is of prime concern. In societies like India where early marriage is still practiced, age at marriage is seemingly less as compared to developed countries like U.S. Marriage pattern also affects fertility as it may lead to either unavailability of marriage partners or can lead to hereditary diseases that can affect both mother and infant. Widowhood in many communities is like social curse and the norms related to it are strictly followed like prohibition of remarriage, life of celibacy etc. that lead to fertility loss (Roth, 2004). Some of the direct factors like use of contraceptive pill, fecundity, adolescent sterility, abortions and age at menopause, education and infanticides terminate fertility (Kayastha, 2007). Mortality among the infants due to gender disparity is still in many areas mostly in India. All factors such as biological, socio-economic and socio-cultural, are responsible for the high mortality rate of children (Das and Das, 2015).

Materials and Methods

Village Profile

The present study was conducted among the women of Vadabalija community (fishing community) in Annavaram village of Andhra Pradesh from 15th December, 2015 to 5th January, 2016. Annavaram village is located 15 km east of Tagarapuvalasa town of Bheemunipatnam mandal of Visakhapatnam district, Andhra Pradesh. The entire village comprises Vada/Vodabalija caste which is a traditional marine fishing community. The village is situated near the banks of the great Bay of Bengal. The village is situated on the sea coast. People of the village are mostly dependent upon ocean for their subsistence and survival. No statistical sampling technique was applied in the selection of individual and household for the present study.

Sample Size

The result is based upon the data collected from 73 women by visiting house to house.

Method of Data Collection

Nature of demographic data collection was based on the parameters suggested by the World Health Organization (1964-1968). Information on age, sex, marital status, occupation, place of birth, place of residence etc. was collected. The fertility and mortality schedules were completed by filling information on the number of conception, number of live births, birth orders, age, sex, marital status of each of the offspring, number of dead children, cause of death, if any, reproductive wastage (abortion and still births) through in depth interview with each of the married women. Special attention was also made to collect data on socio-economic parameters like occupation, household income, household expenditure, educational attainment of household members especially married women, religious affiliation, age at marriage, awareness and adoption of the family planning method etc. The income groups were categorized into three groups, i.e. low income (< Rs. 1000), middle income (Rs. 1000–Rs. 1667) and high income (>Rs. 1667) groups. Educational level of married women was categorized as literate and illiterate.

Statistical Analysis

All the parameters taken were analysed statistically to find out the mean and the standard error. In order to test the level of significance, *t*-test, ANOVA and chi-square test have been used. MS-Excel software was used for all statistical analysis of the present research.

Results

Table 10.1 shows the mean age at marriage and first child birth among males and females of the Annavaram village. It is found that the mean age at marriage was higher among males (23.35±0.58) than females (17.71±0.43). The differences were statistically significant (t = 7.801; p<0.005). Similarly, the mean age at first child birth was also higher in males (24.52±0.7yrs.) than females (19±0.53yrs.). The t-test indicates that the difference between males and females with respect to age at first child was highly significant (t = 6.076; p<0.05). Table 10.2 shows the mean number of the live births and surviving children are 2.72±0.21 and 2.51±0.19 respectively. Table 10.3 shows the adoption of family planning and health care among the women of Annavaram village. It was seen that family planning measures were adopted by most of the mothers of all age groups and they often visited health centre during pregnancy months as well as during delivery time. Table 10.4 shows the frequency of infant mortality, juvenile mortality and reproductive wastage of the study population. Out of 194 live births of the mother of all ages, six live births died before the age of 1 year and two live births died between 1 to 14

Table 10.1: Mean Age at Marriage and First Child Birth among Males and Females of the Annavaram Village

Sex	*Numbers*	*Mean age of Marriage ±SE yrs*	*Mean age at first child birth ±SE yrs*
Male	73	23.35 ±0.58	24.52 ±0.72
Female	73	17.71 ±0.43	19 ±0.53

$t = 7.801$; $df = 142$; $p<0.05$, $t = 6.076$; $df = 142$; $p<0.05$

Source: Author's Study.

Table 10.2: Mean Live Birth and Mean Surviving Children of Women of Annavaram Village

Number of women above 40 years	*Number of live birth children*	*Number of surviving children*	*Mean live birth of children ±SE*	*Mean surviving children ±SE*
25	98	86	2.72±0.21	2.51±0.19

Source: Author's Study.

Table 10.3: Adoption of Family Planning and Health Care among the Women of Annavaram Village

Age group	*No. of mothers*	*Family planning*		*Health centre*	
		Yes	No	Yes	No
≤19	2	–	2	2	–
20-24	13	5	8	12	1
>25	58	41	17	42	16

Source: Author's Study.

Table 10.4: Infant Mortality, Juvenile Mortality and Reproductive Wastage

Parameters	*Frequency*
Number of mothers	73
Total number of pregnancies	211
Number of live births	194
Number of deaths below 1 year	6
Number of deaths between 1 to 14 years	2
Infant mortality rate	3.09%
Juvenile mortality rate %	1.03%
Total Number of reproductive wastage	7
Reproductive wastage %	3.31%

Source: Author's Study.

years of age. The frequency of the infant and juvenile mortality rate was 3.09 per cent and 1.03 per cent respectively. It indicates that mortality rate especially infant mortality is little high than juvenile mortality in this population. Table further indicates that the rate of reproductive wastage out of total pregnancies was 3.31 per cent. Table 10.5 shows the mean live birth and surviving children by the income level of the household. The mean live birth (2.68±0.19) was found slightly higher in high income family followed by middle income family (2.66±0.20) and low income family (2.65±0.19). The differences in the mean live births in different income levels were statistically significant ($f = 3.19$; $p<0.05$). However, the frequency of mean surviving children was found the same in both low income family (2.47±0.17) and middle income family (2.47±0.18). The high frequency of the mean surviving children (2.49±0.18) was found among the females belonging to the higher income family. Table 10.6 shows the infant mortality rate by the income level of the family. The frequency of infant mortality rate was slightly higher among the middle income family (6.66%) than low income group (2.04%).

Table 10.5: Fertility Rate by Income Level of the Family of Annavaram Village

Income	*Number of mothers*	*Number of live births*	*Number of surviving children*	*Mean live births ±SE*	*Mean surviving children ±SE*
Low	31	98	94	2.65±0.19	2.47±0.17
Middle	24	60	51	2.66±0.20	2.47±0.18
High	18	36	36	2.68±0.19	2.49±0.18

$f= 3.19$; $p<0.05$ (live birth) $f= 3.98$; $p<0.05$ (surviving children)
Source: Author's Study.

Table 10.6: Infant Mortality Rate by Income Level of Family of Annavaram Village

Income	*Number of live births*	*Number of infants*	*Infant mortality*
Low	98	2	2.04%
Middle	60	4	6.66%
High	36	0	–

$\chi^2 = 3.780$; $df= 2$; $p>0.05$
Source: Author's Study.

Discussion

Both fertility and mortality is affected by various factors be it socio-economic factor, biological as well as environmental factor. With the dynamic social change, development programmes, migration, urbanization, accessibility of medical facilities etc., there has been decrease in both fertility and mortality. In 2008, an estimated 3,58,000 women died due to conditions related to pregnancy or childbearing, i.e. maternal conditions (WHO and others, 2010). Most of the parts in south India approached replacement fertility levels and majority of the States had moderate fertility levels while the central States continued to have high level of fertility by 1991 (Martine *et al.*, 1998). The striking features of reproductive change in India are the enormous regional differences in the timing and pace of fertility decline. Education, occupation and income have a key role to play in the socio-economic field that affects fertility and mortality (Dey and Goswami, 2009). Age at marriage is also a vital determinant of fertility rate among the women and thus could directly influence the supply of children (Samola *et al.*, 2006). Women married at earlier age experience longer period of reproductive span and usually have more children. The age at which female get married or first time steps towards the reproductive period of her life has a great impact on fertility. The age at marriage is affected by various factors like the education of women, the cultural beliefs and practices, society women belongs to, status of women etc. The age at marriage differs among different groups of people (Angeles, 2010; Bharathi, 2014). Female age at marriage can also be regarded as the powerful indicator of the status of women. Early marrying of female population shows low female autonomy in the society.

Female education is well-known to be of primary importance for child survival, as well as fertility (Repetto, 1979, 1986; Schultz, 1978; Waldmann, 1992; WHO, 1999). Educated women have other sources of prestige and fulfilment besides reproductive performance (Dyson and Moore, 1983; Cain, 1984). However, it is also argued with the fact that education of women alone does not give all the rights of decision-making to women, but the autonomy of women in the society depends upon the autonomy provided by her culture (Kaufmann and Cleland, 1994). Education level has strong affects on health behaviours and attitudes of individuals (Leone, 2013). Educated women tend to be more aware of the maternal health, nutrition, health and hygiene of her children (Marthi *et al.*, 1995). Educated women are most likely to adopt the contraceptive measures for the betterment of their children in terms of health, education and proper look after. Illiterate women are more introverts and shy and do now follow up the contraceptive measures, which are recommended unless there are some incentives provided. Because of poor connectivity, lack of awareness, inadequate and poorly functional infrastructure, rural poor have inadequate access to basic minimum services which affects their overall health.

Based on the data collected during the fieldwork among 73 Vadabalija women, it is found that the mean age at marriage is higher among the males than females and the differences in the mean age at marriage values are statistically significant. The mean age at first child birth is also higher among males than females which are also found highly significant. In both the findings, the possible reason may be because of the practice of early marriage among girl child. Less differences is seen between the live birth and number of surviving children among women who have attained 40 years and above which indicates that the mortality rate among the children is less. Family planning methods were adopted by most of the women in the village of all age groups and health care centre were visited by most of the women during pre-to-post pregnancy. This may be because of the health care awareness programmes conducted by ANM nurses in collaboration with ICDS centre in the village, initiatives from the government health sectors that emphasizes on small and healthy family, the incentives given for undergoing through family planning measures or due to work pressure, as most of the household works are performed by women. Infant mortality is slightly higher than juvenile mortality because of the poor socio-economic condition that confines them to provide required goods in terms of better nutrition and better health care. It also could be due to limited time for mothers to look after their infants as they are busy most of the time engaging in household chores and other activities. In case of grown up children, they can somehow manage to survive and look after themselves. The mean live birth is more or less the same in the higher income, middle income and low income group. Similarly, the mean surviving children also found more or less the same in the higher income, middle income and low income family. Study has shown that economic condition influences the fertility rate to a large extent (Dey and Goswami, 2009). The frequency of infant mortality rate was found higher among the low income and illiterate mothers in the present study. The reason could be due to better nutrition, medical facilities and health care which can easily afford by the higher income family than low income family.

This study is a part of dissertation in which the duration of fieldwork was time bound. Communication also plays an important role in field research. It is not always possible to get the exact and said data through an interpreter. Also, the study accounts the data of one fishing community. However, the study is important as it gives close insights of the fertility and mortality status. It is also useful in understanding the impacts and importance of secondary sources for public health in general. In one hand, the decreasing fertility due to socio-economic and socio-cultural factors shows loss of fertility even if the fecundity is high and in another hand the decreasing mortality (especially infant mortality) shows improvement in health care system. The study also shows the role of external sources, i.e. media, health care programmes in spreading the health care messages in mass. The study helps in knowing the present situation of the population, their general and genuine needs which are given less importance. Although family planning has become common in this community and it is in a way good as the parents can provide basic needs to their children if they are few yet it is also an obligation to undergo family planning due to poor socio-economic status. This in terms of public health, the initiative of government or other concerned departments should not only focus on making them ready for small families, but should also see what are the other necessary steps that can be taken or needed for better heath in general.

Conclusion

The present study among the Vadabalija women of Annavaram village highlights poor socio-economic conditions, early marriage and low education of girl child, preference of male child etc. that has affected both fertility and mortality. Female literacy is low as compared to male because of the early marriage of girl child. Another factor for the decrease in female literacy is, after the completion of secondary schooling most girls do not or are not allowed to opt for higher studies as there are no higher secondary schools in the village and one need to go far away from the village to attend higher education.

Early marriage is also common among the female child of this village. However, it is seen that female child is not considered burden but blessings especially because they help in the house hold chores and also because the concept of dowry was not present in this society until recent years. Now, the preference of male child is only due to the dowry. Nevertheless, both male and female child is equally loved by their parents.

Family planning measures (sterilization, mostly of women) is seen to be very common that has led in the decrease in fertility even if the fecundity is high. Women are engaged in almost all kinds of household activities. In few cases women suffered from miscarriage caused due to heavy duty tasks like fetching water. The study also shows that there has been strong initiative taken by the concerned department that has brought about a sense of health care among the people especially among the mother and other expecting and married women. However, it is not just the initiative from the secondary sources but also the individual's decisions and steps that counts when it comes to family planning and healthcare during pre-and post-delivery of the child.

The mortality of children is seen especially among families who cannot afford the expenses of medical facilities and also those who are illiterate. It is observed that such families are focused more into traditional methods for curing diseases which are cheap, but sometimes not effective. The result shows that socio-economic condition of the family plays important roles on determining health. Better education and family income tend to have better yet controlled fertility (implementation of contraceptive measures), better health care of both child and mother where as it also shows the decrease in child mortality.

To conclude, the study of fertility and mortality status not just gives the idea of population and health of a population group, but also throws light on the different aspects like social change, the initiatives from different sources for public health etc. which are responsible for the differential fertility and mortality rates.

Acknowledgements

I take this opportunity to thank many people for their direct and indirect contribution towards the completion of this research paper. Firstly, I would like to express my sincere gratitude to Dr. K.R. Rama Mohan, Department Head and Dr. Maibam Samson Singh, Assistant Professor, Department of Anthropology, Sikkim University, without their immense support this work would not have been possible. I am truly thankful to all the other faculty members of Department of Anthropology, Sikkim University, for their valuable help and advices. I would like to express my appreciation to all the interpreters and the entire villagers of Annavaram for being co-operative and helpful during the fieldwork. Lastly, I express my sincere gratitude to my beloved family and friends for their continuous support and encouragement.

References

Angeles, L. (2010). "Demographic transition: Analyzing the effect on fertility and mortality", *Journal of Population Ecology*, 23: 99-120.

Bharathi, K. (2014). "Impact on consanguinity on fertility and mortality", *Journal of Humanities and Social Science*, 19(4): 39-42.

Cain, M. (1984). "Women's status and fertility in developing countries: Son preference and economic security", *World Bank Staff Working Papers*, 682.

Das, N.K. and Das, R. (2015). "A study on cause of death among the tribal children of Udalguri District, Assam", *International Journal Medical Science Public Health*, 4: 1060-1065.

Dey, S. and Goswami, S. (2009). "Fertility pattern and its correlates in North East India", *Journal of Human Ecology*, 26(2):145-152.

Dyson, T. and Moore, M. (1983). "On kinship structure, female autonomy and demographic behaviour in India", *Population and Development Review*, 9(1):35-60.

Heuveline, P. (2003). *Mortality and Fertility Interaction: New Insights from Recent Population Dynamics in Cambodia*, http://www.prgs.edu/content/dam/rand/www/external/labor/seminars/adp/pdfs/adpheuveline.pdf (Accessed on 5 April, 2016).

Kapoor, A.K., Kshatriya, G.K. and Kapoor, S. (2003). "Fertility and mortality differential among the population group of Himalayas", *Human Biology*, 75(5):729-747.

Kaufmann, G. and Cleland, J. (1994). "Maternal education and child survival: Anthropological response to demographic evidence", *Health Transition Review*, 4(2):196-199.

Kayastha, S.L. (2007). *Geography of Population*, New Delhi: Rawat Publication.

Leone, S. (2013). *Sierra Leone Demographic and Health Survey*. http://dhsprogram.com/pubs/pdf/PR42.pdf (Accessed on 23 April, 2016).

Marthi, M., Guio, A.N. and Dreze, J. (1995). "Mortality, fertility and gender biased in India: A district level analysis", *Population and Development Review*, 21(4):745-782.

Martine, G., Gupta, M.D. and Chen, L.C. (1998). *Reproductive Change in India and Brazil,* New Delhi: Oxford University Press.

Notestein, F.W. (1945). "Population: The long view", In: Schultz, T.W. (ed.) *Food for the World,* Chicago: Chicago University Press.

Reddy, K.S.N. and Sudha, F. (2010). "Factors affecting fertility and mortality: A case study among the Setti Balija community of Andhra Pradesh", *Anthropologist*, 12(4):271-275.

Repetto, R. (1979). "The interaction of fertility and the size distribution of income: A comment", *Journal of Development Studies*, 16.

Repetto, R. (1986). "Soil loss and population pressure in Java", *Ambio*, 15(1):14 18.

Roth, E.A. (2004). *Culture, Biology and Anthropological Demography,* New York: Cambridge University Press.

Samola, T.D., Nabhakumar, W. and Jibonkumar, S. (2006). "Fertility study among the ithing of Manipur, India", *The Internet Journal of Biological Anthropology*, 1(1).

Schultz, T.P. (1978). "Fertility and child mortality over the life cycle: Aggregate and individual evidence", *The American Economic Review*, 68(2):208-215.

Waldmann, R.J. (1992). "Income distribution and infant mortality", *The Quarterly Journal of Economics*, 107(4):1283-1302.

WHO (1999). *The World Health Report 1999: Making a Difference.* Geneva: WHO Press.

WHO (2010). *Trends in Maternal Mortality: 1990 to 2008*—Estimates developed by WHO, UNICEF, UNFPA and The World Bank. Geneva: WHO Press.

11

A Study on Segregation Distortion of ABO and Rh(D) Blood Group and Reproductive Performance in Bengali Population

Diptendu Chatterjee, Pranabesh Sarkar, Arup Ratan Bandyopadhyay and *Moumita Sadhukhan*

Introduction

The ABO blood groups are studied first and considerable detail because these were the first human blood groups being discovered and still the most important. Moreover, the techniques involved in their estimation from the basic of almost all blood grouping methods, those used for other blood group system being to a large extent modifier using different reagents media ones temperatures of reaction. Since the publication of Daniels (2002) the problem concerning the elimination of blood group genes had been the subject matter of a number of scientists. Levine and Rosenfield (1961) have provided a highly critical appraisal on the subject. In later years Boorman (1967), Mange (1997), Rosenfield (1973), Mourant (1976), Clegg (1979), Weine (1943) have updated the observations on the matter. Three principles but mutually exclusive mechanism, namely mortality of the genotypes (Mourant, 1947; Ford, 1940; Hosoi, 2008; Ragan, 2000; Takano, 1972; Clarke, 1972; Schaap, 1984; Bottini, 2001; Malekasgar, 2004), distortion of different blood groups (Sono, 2009; Bandyopadhyay, 2011; Mohanty, 2010; Pourjafari, 2004; Marsh, 1090) and differential fertility of different genotypes (Bandyopadhyay, 2011; Badet, 1976; Lloyd, 1968; Race, 1968; Shen, 1968; Watkins, 1959; Yoshida, 1982; Ogunbsi, 2007) were thought to be responsible (Richon, 1970; Scid, 2000; Gao, 2009; Marwaha,

2012) for the maintenance of polymorphism in blood groups especially of the ABO system. Selection due to feto-maternal incompatibility with regard to the ABO and Rh blood groups causing HDN of the new born (Levine *et al.*, 1961) although initially was found to be a powerful agent for incompatibility selection (Bandyopadhyay, 2011), but in later years was found to have some protective effective heterozygotic elimination due to interaction between the ABO and Rh incompatibility (Levine, 1961). It is, however, yet to be thoroughly known whether a similar type of protection is offered against the incompatibility selection in the form of differential fertility ad foetal wastage due to incompatibility mating status of the couple. Distortion of segregation ratio in blood group among the offspring is accounted as one of the unequivocal evidence of system in uterus; more ones it is also indicative of prezygotic selection; i.e. preferential transmission of certain gametes carrying ABO gene, which has been referred to as mitotic drive (Bandyopadhyay, 2011). Distortion of segregation ratio in the form of deficiency of an offspring in mating between 'O' mother and 'A' father was firmly noted by Mohammed, 2012, Bandyopadhyay, 2011, accounted it as due to ABO incompatibility selection in uterus. This was later on found to be applicable also to other six types of ABO incompatibility mating (Morgan, 1969; Lorigan, 2000). In subsequent years in most of the studies on ABO incompatibility foetal was found to be much higher among 'O' group mothers than mothers belonging to the other groups (Berberrovic, 2004). In International samples with Omu (1998), Bakkeheim (2009), Guleria (2007), Nasseri (2006). Working with Indian subjects Bandyopadhyay *et al.* (2011) and many other scholars. In view of the above mentioned fact is the present study Reproductive Performance of Bengali Caste population on the basis of ABO blood group in a set of data comprising individuals including off-springs and parents were studied to find out to what extent the incompatibility selection could cause the segregation distortion of ABO blood group and thereby bring inconsistency in the distribution of genotypes between parents and off-springs.

The objective of the present study is to observe the reproductive performance of Bengali Hindu Caste population on the basis of ABO and Rh (D) blood group.

Materials and Methods

The present study has been carried out among the Bengali families of Metropolis Kolkata along with North 24 Parganas, Hooghly. 141 apparently healthy married couples and their offsprings and total number of participants were 497, have been considered for this cross-sectional study in the metropolitan area of Kolkata. Data for the present study has been collected by using specially prepared and pre-tested schedule. Blood group has been determined by using the conventional method (Boorman and Dodd, 1967). Then data has been checked and computed accordingly. Analysis was done by using the Microsoft Office, 2007. For selection of participants only Hindu Bengali caste family considered here, and there is no age effect on blood group only considered the generations.

Results and Discussion

In the present study the total numbers of participants were 497, where, 282 numbers of participants are from Parental generation and 215 numbers of subjects are from offspring generation. In 282 numbers of subjects of parental generation there are each 141 number of subjects of male and female. And between 215 numbers of subjects of offspring generation, 90 are males and 125 are females. Between the studied populations the numbers of offsprings are 215, between which 90 are male and 125 are female. The mean birth weight of male and female is 8.29 kg and 7.87 kg. The mean birth weight of first baby generations, second baby generations and third baby generations are 2.66, 2.65, and 2.71 respectively whether it was male or female. In between 2.61, 2.77 and 2.91 are mean birth weight of male offspring. And 2.69, 2.57 and 2.61 are mean birth weight of female offspring. In present studied population when it is considered the Socio-economic status with Educational and Economical parameters, then it was observed that for the educational status the majority of my studied population is Graduates with 71 and 57 numbers of subjects in both case of male and female. Then it leads to higher secondary level in both parental generations with 28 and 39 in number and its frequency 19.85 per cent and 27.65 per cent. Next there is a twist is observed in parental generations, where the third major position of educational status of male is University with 19 numbers of subjects carrying 13.47 per cent, for female it is

Madhyamik level education with 30 numbers of subjects carrying 21.27 per cent. And the fourth major position of educational status is for male *Madhyamik* level with 18 numbers of subjects carrying 12.76 per cent and for female it is University level with 13 numbers of subjects carrying 9.21 per cent. The last majority is literate in case of both male and female with 5 and 2 numbers of subjects carrying 3.54 per cent and 1.41 per cent respectively. Considering Economic status of studied Bengali caste population's family leads by below Rs. 20,000 per month, then below Rs. 30,000 per month, after that above Rs. 30,000 per month and lastly the below Rs. 10,000 per month earning family.

In parental generation, there are 52, 11, 71, 7 are Phenotype of O, A, B and AB blood groups respectively of male parental generation, which covers the 36.87 per cent, 7.80 per cent, 50.35 per cent, 4.96 per cent of studied population respectively. And they have allele frequency of p, q, r are 0.06, 0.34, 0.60. And also there are 32, 30, 73, 13 are Phenotype of O, A, B and AB blood groups respectively of female parental generation, which covers the 22.69 per cent, 21.27 per cent, 51.77 per cent, 4.25 per cent of studied population respectively. And they have allele frequency of p, q, r are 0.19, 0.35, 0.53. In offspring generations, there are 34, 12, 43, 1 are Phenotype of O, A, B and AB blood groups respectively of male offspring generation, which covers the 37.77 per cent, 13.33 per cent, 47.77 per cent, 1.11 per cent of studied population. And they have allele frequency of p, q, r are 0.11, 0.29, 0.60. And there are 38, 18, 66, 3 are Phenotype of O, A, B and AB blood groups respectively of male parental generation, which covers the 30.4 per cent, 14.4 per cent, 52.8 per cent, 2.4 per cent of studied population. And they have allele frequency of p, q, r are 0.29, 0.34, 0.37. In our studied population, between 231 male numbers of subjects, O Blood group are 86, which covers the 37.22 per cent of studied population. A Blood group are 23, which covers the 9.95 per cent of studied population. B Blood group are 114, which covers the 49.35 per cent of studied population and AB Blood groups are in 8, which covers the 3.46 per cent of studied population And between 266 female number of subjects, O Blood group is 70, which covers the 26.31 per cent of studied population A Blood group is 48, which covers the 18.04 per cent of studied population B blood group is

139, which covers the 52.25 per cent of studied population and AB blood groups are in 9, which covers the 3.38 per cent of studied population.

In parental generation, there are 130, 11 Rh(D)+ and Rh(D)– blood groups respectively of male parental generation, which covers the 92.19 per cent, 7.80 per cent of studied population respectively. And they have allele frequency of D and d are 0.92, 0.08. And also there are 133, 8 Rh(D)+ and Rh(D)–blood groups respectively of female parental generation, which covers the 94.32 per cent, 5.60 per cent of studied population respectively. And they have allele frequency of D and d are 0.94, 0.06. In offspring generation, there are 88, 2 Rh(D)+ and Rh(D)–blood groups respectively of male offspring generation, which covers 97.77 per cent, 2.22 per cent of studied population respectively. And they have allele frequency of D and d are 0.97, 0.03. And also there are 116, 9 Rh(D)+ and Rh(D)– blood groups respectively of female offspring generation, which covers the 92.80 per cent, 7.20 per cent of studied population respectively. And they have allele frequency of D and d are 0.92, 0.08.

In the studied Bengali caste population, it has been observed that couple combinations with regard to both the ABO and Rh(D) Blood groups. In between ABO compatible combination observed in 102 pairs, between them 96 are in Rh(D) compatible combination and 6 are in Rh(D) incompatible combination. The frequency of ABO compatible–Rh(D) compatible combination is 94.11 per cent and ABO compatible–Rh(D) incompatible combination is 5.88 per cent. And in between ABO incompatible combination observed in 39 pairs, between them 37 are in Rh(D) compatible combination and 2 are in Rh(D) incompatible combination. The frequency of ABO incompatible–Rh(D) compatible combination is 94.87 per cent and ABO incompatible–Rh(D) incompatible combination is 5.12 per cent. And where Rh(D) compatible–ABO compatible the frequency is 72.18 per cent. Rh(D) compatible–ABO incompatible the frequency is 27.81 per cent. Rh(D) incompatible–ABO compatible the frequency is 75 per cent. Rh(D) incompatible–ABO incompatible the frequency is 25 per cent. It can be observed that the Segregation of ABO blood groups among the Children according to the Compatible mating types of parents, In O-O mother-father combinations total parity is 13, which gives 19 offsprings are of O blood group. The frequency of O blood group offspring is 100 per cent.

Then in A-O mother-father combinations total parity is 15, which gives 14 offsprings are of O blood group. The frequency of O blood group offspring is 58.33 per cent and 10 offsprings are of A blood group. The frequency of A blood group offspring is 41.66 per cent. In B-O mother-father combinations total parity is 22, which gives 17 offsprings are of O blood group. The frequency of O blood group offspring is 44.73 per cent and 21 offsprings are of B blood group. The frequency of B blood group offspring is 55.26 per cent. Again in AB-O mother-father combination's total parity is 2, which gives 1 offspring of O blood group. The frequency of O blood group offspring is 33.33 per cent and 2 offsprings are of B blood group. The frequency of B blood group offspring is 66.66 per cent. In A-A mother-father combination's total parity is 1, which gives 3 offsprings are of A blood groups. The frequency of A blood group offspring is 100 per cent. Among B-B mother-father combination's total parity is 45, which gives 6 offsprings are of O blood group. The frequency of O blood group offspring is 9.09 per cent and 1 offsprings are of A blood group. The frequency of A blood group offspring is 1.51 per cent and 59 offsprings are of B blood group. The frequency of B blood group offspring is 89.39 per cent. In AB-AB mother-father combination's total parity is 0. Between AB-A mother-father combination's total parity is 1, which gives 1 offspring of A blood group. The frequency of A blood group offspring is 100 per cent. Lastly in AB-B mother-father combinations total parity is 3, which gives 1 offsprings are of O blood group. The frequency of O blood group offspring is 25 per cent and 2 offsprings are of B blood group. The frequency of B blood group offspring is 50 per cent and 1 offsprings are of AB blood group. The frequency of AB blood group offspring is 25 per cent. Finally the Compatible couple combinations wise frequencies are 12.74 per cent, 14.78 per cent, 21.56 per cent, 1.96 per cent, 0.98 per cent, 44.11 per cent, 0 per cent, 0.98 per cent and 2.94 per cent out of 102 number of subjects. Again, it can be observed that the segregation of ABO blood groups among the children according to the incompatible mating types of parents. In O-A mother-father combination's total parity is 5, which gives 5 offsprings are of O blood group. The frequency of O blood group offspring is 83.33 per cent and 1 offspring of A blood group. The frequency of A blood group offspring is 16.66 per cent. In O-B mother-father combination's total parity is 13, which gives 10 offsprings are of O blood group. The frequency of O blood group offspring is 43.47 per cent and 13 offsprings are of B blood group. The frequency of B blood group offspring is 56.52 per cent. Again in O-AB mother-father combination's total parity is 1, which gives 2 offsprings are of A blood group. The frequency of A blood group offspring is 100 per cent. In B-A mother-father combination's total parity is 4, which gives 1 offspring of O blood group. The frequency of O blood group offspring 20 per cent and 1 offspring of A blood group. The frequency of A blood group offspring is 20 per cent and 2 offsprings are of B blood group. The frequency of B blood group offspring is 40 per cent and 1 offsprings are of AB blood group. The frequency of AB blood group is 20 per cent. Among A-B mother-father combination's total parity is 10, which gives 5 offsprings are of A blood group. The frequency of A blood group offspring is 35.71 per cent and 7 offsprings are of B blood group. The frequency of B blood group offspring is 50 per cent and 2 offsprings are of AB blood group. The frequency of AB blood group offspring is 14.28 per cent. Between A-AB mother-father combinations total parity is 4, which gives 5 offsprings are of A blood group. The frequency of A blood group offspring is 71.42 per cent and 2 offsprings are of B blood group. The frequency of B blood group offspring is 28.57 per cent. At last in B-AB mother-father combination's total parity is 2, which gives 1 offspring of A blood group. The frequency of A blood group offspring is 33.33 per cent and 2 offsprings are of B blood group. The frequency of B blood group offspring is 66.66 per cent. Finally, the incompatible couple combination-wise frequencies are 12.82 per cent, 33.33 per cent, 2.56 per cent, 10.25 per cent, 25.64 per cent, 10.25 per cent, and 5.12 per cent out of 39 number of subjects. It was observed that the segregation of 'O' and 'Non-O' blood groups among children in reciprocal O and Non-O (A/B/AB) mating types, have the 39 number of couples, when mothers are of Non O and fathers are of O type, then the Blood group of children are 32 O type and 33 Non-O type. And 19 number of couples, where mothers are O type and Fathers are Non-O type.

Among Reproductive performance and foetal wastage by mating status of the couples, total number of ABO compatible pregnancies are 184 in number among them 157 are living children its frequency is 85.32 per cent, 25 are neo-natal death its frequency 13.58 per cent and 2 are post-natal death, its frequency 1.08 per cent. Between them total pregnancy wastage is 27 in number and its frequency is 14.67 per cent. Total number of ABO incompatible pregnancies are 77 in number among them 61 are living children its frequency is 79.22 per cent, 14 are neo-natal deaths its frequency 18.18 per cent and 2 are post-natal death, its frequency 2.59 per cent. Between them total pregnancy wastage is 16 in number and its frequency is 20.77 per cent. Again among Reproductive performance and foetal wastage by mating status of the couples, total number of Rh(D) compatible pregnancies are 175 in number among them 141 are living children it's frequency is 80.57 per cent, 30 are neo-natal death its frequency 17.14 per cent and 4 post-natal death, its frequency 2.28 per cent. Between them total pregnancy wastages were 34 in number and its frequency is 19.42 per cent. Total number of Rh(D) incompatible pregnancies are 18 in number among them 16 are living children its frequency is 88.88 per cent, 2 are neo-natal death its frequency 11.11 per cent. Between them total pregnancy wastages were 2 in number and its frequency is 25 per cent. The present study has done on the basis of family study for the segregation analysis. Distribution of ABO blood groups and their gene frequencies among 215 number of offsprings and their parents are seen. No heterogeneity in distribution of blood groups among the parents is found. Data of the parental generation were combined together and when compared with their children, difference in the distribution of blood groups between parents and children was observed. This was due to increase of gene with simultaneous decrease of p and q genes among the children compared to those among their parents (Nasseri, 2006; Kneib, 2002; Wallerstein, 1949; Wikman, 2007; Lurie, 1998; Mamouri, 2002; Sarici, 2002; Thilo, 2007; Bandyopadhyay *et al.*, 2011). Segregation of ABO blood group among the children classified according to ABO compatible and ABO incompatible mating types of their parents has been presented here. Frequencies of 'A' and 'B' children are found to be lower in incompatible mating types than those in children born in compatible ones. Frequencies of 'O' Blood group children remaining almost same in both categories of the parental generation. In segregation of 'O' blood group and Non-'O' (A/B/AB) blood group, among the children born reciprocal 'O' blood group and Non-'O' (A/B/AB) mating types, distortion was evident. Significant increase of Non-'O' offspring and decrease of 'O' offspring was noted in compatible mating (Non-'O' mother and 'O' father). An opposite picture was noted among the children born compatible ('O' mother and Non-'O' father) mating where decrease of Non-'O' children and excess of 'O' children could be seen. Moreover, deficiency of Non-'O' blood group (A/B/AB) children relative to 'O' blood group children in compatible mating compared to those in compatible ones. Deficiencies of A and B children relative to O children in mating between O mother and A and B father were compared with those children derived out of mating. Levine and Rosenfield (1973) by using cross ratio (r) and significant of ratio (r) was tested by using chi-square. The obtained result of the present study was compared with those derived from as number of authors like Bandyopadhyay *et al.* (2011). Levine and Rosenfield (1961) computed a general deficiency of incompatible offspring born to O mother as when data of all authors, mostly working on European population was computed. Different noteworthy work on Indian population was also considered here. Combining all those data obtained from studies of Indian authors significant deficiency of in A 3 and B 13 children born to O mother were found. The total deficiency of A and B incompatible children among O mother was found to be 16 compared to deficiency as reported by Rosenfield, (1973) and Bandyopadhyay *et al.* (2011). Out of the several factors which might be at work for the causation of such types of deficiencies in the incompatibility in the incompatibility selection between ABO and Rh(D) blood groups, protective interaction of ABO incompatibility against Rh(D) sensitization, and increasing use of anti-D gamma globulin in Rh(D) incompatibility might have produced some beneficial effect against the Rh(D) sensitization and elimination of the incompatibility heterozygous. The segregation distortion in each generation may cause the change in genetic make up and incompatibility might be the cause of fetal wastage. So, it might be the cause of change in gene frequency in one population. It might be a vital public health issue. The above mentioned fact could be well understood by the fact that quantum of reproductive performance and foetal wastage as found among the couples with incompatible in both the ABO and Rh(D) systems do not differ significantly from those of the couples having compatible in ABO and incompatible in Rh(D) systems. It will thus be apparent from the forging presentation that there exists definite evidence for distortion in segregation ratio of ABO blood groups among their children caused by deficiency of incompatible genotypes due to heterozygote selection. Elimination of incompatible genotypes as expected brought significant inconsistency in the distribution of ABO blood groups between parents and children.

Table 11.1: Distribution of Population

	Male	*Female*	*Total*
Parental generation	141	141	282
Offspring generation	90	125	215
Total	**231**	**266**	**497**

Source: Author's Study.

Table 11.2: Description and General Overview of Offspring Generation

	Number	*Male*	*Female*	*Mean Birth Weight*	*Mean birth weight of male*	*Mean birth weight of female*
Baby-1	141	59	82	2.66	2.61	2.69
Baby-2	63	24	39	2.65	2.77	2.57
Baby-3	11	7	4	2.71	2.91	2.61
Total	**215**	**90**	**125**	**8.02**	**8.29**	**7.87**

Baby 1 mean 1st parity, 2 mean 2nd and 3 mean 3rd.
Source: Author's Study.

Table 11.3(a): Educational Status of Parental Generations

Education	*Literate*	*Madhyamik Level*	*Higher Secondary level*	*College*	*University*	*Total*
Male	5	18	28	71	19	141
%	3.54	12.76	19.85	50.35	13.47	
Female	2	30	39	57	13	141
%	1.41	21.27	27.65	40.42	9.21	

Source: Author's Study.

Justification of such table: Education might the cause of intercaste marriage, it might be one of the determinants of the segregation distortion.

Table 11.3(b): Family Income of Parental Generations

Family Income per month	*below 10,000*	*below 20,000*	*below 30,000*	*above 30,000*	*Total family*
	25 17.73	47 33.33	43 30.49	26 18.43	141

Source: Author's Study.

Justification: Income might the cause of intercaste marriage, it might be one of the determinants of the segregation distortion.

Table 11.4: Distribution of Blood Group in Parental Generation

Blood Group	*A*	*B*	*AB*	*O*
Male	11	71	7	52
Female	30	73	6	32

N = 141 each male and female.
Source: Author's Study.

Table 11.5: Distribution of Population among First Parity (Baby)

Blood Group	*A*	*B*	*AB*	*O*
Male	8	28	1	22
Female	11	45	3	23

N = 141 including Male = 59, Female = 82
Source: Author's Study.

Table 11.6: Distribution of Population among Second Parity (Baby)

Blood Group	*A*	*B*	*AB*	*O*
Male	3	12	0	9
Female	6	18	0	15

N = 63 including Male = 24, Female = 39
Source: Author's Study.

Table 11.7: Distribution of Population among Third Parity (Baby)

Blood Group	*A*	*B*	*AB*	*O*
Male	1	3	0	3
Female	1	3	0	0

N = 11 including Male = 7, Female = 4
Source: Author's Study.

Table 11.8: Distribution of ABO Blood Group and Allele Frequencies of Parental Generation

	Phenotype				*Total*	*Allele Frequency*		
	O	*A*	*B*	*AB*	*N*	*P*	*q*	*r*
Male	52	11	71	7	141	0.06	0.34	0.6
%	36.87	7.80	50.35	4.96				
Female	32	30	73	6	141	0.19	0.35	0.46
%	22.69	21.27	51.77	4.25				
Total	**84**	**41**	**144**	**13**	**282**	**0.13**	**0.34**	**0.53**
%	**29.78**	**14.53**	**51.06**	**4.60**				

Chi-square value = 13.6; when df = 5.
Source: Author's Study.

Table 11.9: Distribution of ABO Blood Group and Allele Frequencies of Offspring Generation

	Phenotype				*Total*	*Allele Frequency*		
	O	A	B	AB	N	P	q	r
Male	34	12	43	1	90	0.11	0.29	0.60
%	37.77	13.33	47.77	1.11				
Female	38	18	66	3	125	0.29	0.34	0.37
%	30.4	14.4	52.8	2.4				
Total	**72**	**30**	**109**	**4**	**215**	**0.32**	**0.32**	**0.36**
%	**33.48**	**13.95**	**50.69**	**1.86**				

Chi-square value = 11.24; when df = 5.
Source: Author's Study.

Table 11.10: Distribution of ABO Blood group and allele frequencies of all participants (Pooled)

	Phenotype				*Total*	*Allele Frequency*		
	O	A	B	AB	N	P	q	r
Male	86	23	114	8	231	0.08	0.32	0.60
%	37.22	9.95	49.35	3.46				
Female	70	48	139	9	266	0.16	0.34	0.50
%	26.31	18.04	52.25	3.38				
Total	156	71	253	17	497	0.12	0.33	0.55
%	31.38	14.28	50.90	3.42				

Source: Author's Study.

Table 11.11: Distribution of Rh(D) Blood Group and Allele Frequencies in the Parental Generation

	Blood group		*Total*	*Allele frequency*	
	Rh(D)+	*Rh(D)-*	*N*	*D*	*d*
Male	130	11	141	0.92	0.08
%	92.19	7.80			
Female	133	8	141	0.94	0.06
%	94.32	5.60			
Total	**263**	**19**	**282**		
%	**93.26**	**6.70**			

Source: Author's Study.

Table 11.12: Distribution of Rh(D) Blood Group and Allele Frequencies in the Offspring Generation

	Blood group		*Total*	*Allele frequency*	
	Rh(D)+	*Rh(D)-*	*N*	*D*	*d*
Male	88	2	90	0.97	0.03
%	97.77	2.22			
Female	116	9	125	0.92	0.08
%	92.80	7.20			
Total	**204**	**11**	**215**		
%	**94.88**	**5.11**			

Source: Author's Study.

Table 11.13: Couple Combinations with Regard to Both the ABO and Rh(D) Blood Groups

Couple Combination	*Rh(D) Compatible*	*%*	*Rh(D) Incompatible*	*%*	*Total*
ABO Compatible	96	72.18	6	75	102
%	94.11		5.88		
ABO Incompatible	37	27.81	2	25	39
%	94.87		5.12		
Total	**133**	**94.32**	**8**	**5.67**	**141**
%	**94.32**		**5.67**		

Source: Author's Study.

Table 11.14: Segregation of ABO Blood Groups among the Children According to the Compatible Mating Types of Parents

Mating type Compatible		*Total*	*Blood groups of offspring*								*Total number of offsprings*
Mother	*Father*	*N*	*O*	*%*	*A*	*%*	*B*	*%*	*AB*	*%*	
O	O	13	19	100							19
A	O	15	14	58.33	10	41.66					24
B	O	22	17	44.73			21	55.26			38
AB	O	2	1	33.33			2	66.66			3
A	A	1			3	100					3
B	B	45	6	9.09	1	1.51	59	89.39			66
AB	AB										
AB	A	1			1	100					1
AB	B	3	1	25			2	50	1	25	4
Total		**102**	**58**	**36.70**	**15**	**9.49**	**84**	**53.16**	**1**	**0.63**	**158**

Source: Author's Study.

Table 11.15: Segregation of ABO blood groups among the Children according to the incompatible mating types of parents

Mating type Incompatible		*Total*	*Blood groups of offspring*								*Total number of offsprings*
Mother	*Father*	*N*	*O*	*%*	*A*	*%*	*B*	*%*	*AB*	*%*	
O	A	5	5	83.33	1	16.66					6
O	B	13	10	43.47			13	56.52			23
O	AB	1			2	100					2
B	A	4	1	20	1	20	2	40	1	20	5
A	B	10			5	35.71	7	50	2	14.28	14
A	AB	4			5	71.42	2	28.57			7
B	AB	2			1	33.33	2	66.66			3
Total		**39**	**16**	**26.66**	**15**	**25**	**26**	**43.33**	**3**	**5**	**60**

Source: Author's Study.

Table 11.16: Distribution of Couple Combinations in ABO Blood Groups (Mother-Father Combination)

ABO Compatible	*Number*	*%*	*ABO Incompatible*	*Number*	*%*
O-O	13	12.74	O-A	5	12.82
A-O	15	14.78	O-B	13	33.33
B-O	22	21.56	O-AB	1	2.56
AB-O	2	1.96	A-B	10	25.64
A-A	1	0.98	B-A	4	10.25
AB-A	1	0.98	A-AB	4	10.25
B-B	45	44.11	B-AB	2	5.12
AB-B	3	2.94			
AB-AB	0				
Total	**102**		**Total**	**39**	

Source: Author's Study.

Table 11.17: Segregation of 'O' and 'Non-O' Blood Groups among Children in Reciprocal O and Non-O Mating Types.

Mating type		*Number of couple*	*Type*	*Blood group of the children*	
Mother	Father	N		O	Non-O (A/B/AB)
Non-O (A/B/AB)	O	39		32	33
O	Non-O (A/B/AB)	19		15	16

Source: Author's Study.

Table 11.18: Distribution of Reproductive Performance and Foetal Wastage by Mating Status of the Couples

Reproductive performance and foetal wastage	*ABO*		*Rh(D)*	
	Compatible	*Incompatible*	*Compatible*	*Incompatible*
Total number of pregnancies	184	77	175	18
Pregnancy per couple	1.80	1.97	1.31	2.25
Living children	157	61	141	16
%	85.32	79.22	80.57	88.88
Neonatal Death	25	14	30	2
%	13.58	18.18	17.14	11.11
Post-natal Death	2	2	4	
%	1.08	2.59	2.28	
Total pregnancy wastage	27	16	34	2
%	14.67	20.77	19.42	25

Source: Author's Study.

References

Badet, J. (1976). "Serum glycosyltransferase activity associated with antigen biosynthesis in blood groups A and B. Study of normal B group and cis AB group subjects", *Rev. Fr. Transfus. Immunohematol,* 19:105-16.

Bakkeheim, E., Bergerud, U., Schmidt-Melbye AC. (2009). "Maternal IgG anti-A and anti-B titres predict outcome in ABO-incompatibility in the neonate", *ActaPaediatr,*. 98:1896-901.

Bandyopadhyay, A.R., Chatterjee, D., Chatterjee, M. (2011). "Maternal foetal interaction in the ABO System: A comparative analysis of healthy mother and couples with spontaneous abortion in Bengalee population", *Am. J. Hum. Biol.,* 23:76-9.

Berberovic, L., Redzic, A., Sosic, B. (2004). "Impact of ABO blood groups on the fertility of different parental pairs", *Bosn. J. Basic. Med. Sci.,* 4:19-24.

Boorman Kathleen, Ethel, Dodd Barbara, Edith (1967). *An Introduction to Blood Group Serology: Theory, Techniques, Practical Applications* (4th ed), Vol. 67, Boston. Little Brown.

Boorman, K.E., Dodd, B.E. (1966). *An Introduction to Blood Group Serology.* UK. JA Churchill.

Bottini, N., Meloni, G.F., Finocchi, A. (2001). "Maternal-fetal interaction in the ABO system: A comparative analysis of healthy mothers and couples with recurrent spontaneous abortion suggests a protective effect of B incompatibility", *Hum. Biol.,* 73:167-74.

Clarke, C.A. (1972). "Practical effects of blood group incompatibility between mother and fetus", *BMJ.,* 2:90-5.

Clegg, E.J. (1979). "ABO and Rh blood groups in the Outer Hebrides", *Annals of Human Biology,* 6(5): 457-470.

Daniels, G. (2002). *Human Blood Groups*, 2nd edition. USA: Blackwell Science.

Ford, E.B. (1940). "Polymorphism and Taxonomy", In: Huxley, J. (ed). *The New Systematics*. Oxford.

Gao, X.Y., Huang, H., Li LD. (2009). Hemolytic disease of neonates due to anti-M: report of one case and review of reports of 21 cases. *ZhonghuaErKeZaZhi,* 47:648-52.

Guleria, I., Sayegh, M.H. (2007). "Maternal acceptance of the foetus: True human tolerance." *J. Immunol.,* 178:3345-51.

Hosoi, E. (2008). "Biological and clinical aspects of ABO blood group system", *J. Med Invest.,* 55:174-82.

Kneib, M.T., Hamon, I., Miton, A. (2002). "Management of severe neonatal Rh disease following in utero exchange transfusion: Towards a new strategy", *Arch Pediatr.,* 9:1078-82.

Levine, P., Rosenfield, R.E., White, J. (1961). "The first example of the Rh phenotype rGrG." *Am. J. Hum. Genet.,* 13:299-305.

Lloyd, K.O., Kabat, E.A., Licerio, E. (1968). "Immunochemical studies on blood groups. 38 Structures and activities of oligosaccharides produced by alkaline degradation of blood-group Lewis-a substance. Proposed structure of the carbohydrate chains of human blood-group A, B, H, Le-a, and Le-b substances", *Biochemistry,* 7:2976-90.

Lorigan, P.C., Sharma, S., Bright, N. (2000). "Characteristics of women with recurrent molar pregnancies", *Gynecol Oncol.*, 78:288-92.

Lurie, S., Sigler, E., Weissman, A., *et al.* (1998). "Association of the Lewis blood-group phenotype with infertility in women", *Int. J. Fertil Womens Med.*, 43:155 8.

Mange, E.J. and Mange, A.P. (1997). *Basic Human Genetics*, New Delhi: Rastogi Publication.

Marsh, W.L. (1990). "Biological roles of blood group antigens", *Yale J. Biol. Med.*, 63:455-60.

Marwaha, N., Dhawan, H., Thakral, B. (2009). "Severe ABO hemolytic disease of newborn with a positive direct antiglobulin test", *Indian J. Pathol. Microbiol.*, 52: 2 (292).

Mohanty, R. and Das, P.K. (2010). "A search for operation of natural selection in ABO blood groups: Evidences from four ethnic groups of Orissa", *Anthropologist,* 12:1-11.

Mohammad Hassanzadeh-Nazarabadi, Sahar Shekouhi, and Najmeh Seif. (2012). "The incidence of spontaneous abortion in mothers with blood group O compared with other blood types", *Int. J. Mol. Cell. Med.,* 1(2): 99-104.

Morgan, W.T., Watkins, W.M. (1969). "Genetic and biochemical aspects of human blood-group A-, B-, H-, Le-a-and Le-b-specificity", *Br. Med. Bull.*, 25:30-4.

Mourant, A.E., Kopec, A.C. (1976). *The distribution of the human blood groups and other polymorphisms*. London: Oxford University Press.

Mourant, A.E. (1974). "The use of blood groups in anthropology", *The Journal of the Royal Anthropological Institute of Great Britain and Ireland,* 77: 139 144.

Regan, L., Rai, R. (2000). "Epidemiology and the medical causes of miscarriage", *Best Pract. Res. Cl. Ob.*, 4:839-54.

Nasseri, F., Mamouri, G.A., Babaei, H. (2006). "Intravenous immunoglobulin in ABO and Rh hemolytic diseases of newborn", *Saudi Med. J.*, 27:1827-30.

Ogunlesi, T.A., Dedeke, I.O., Adekanmbi, A.F. (2007). "The incidence and outcome of bilirubin encephalopathy in Nigeria: A bi-centre study", *Niger J. Med.*, 16:354-9.

Omu AE, Al-Mutawa M, Al-Qattan F. (1998). "ABO blood group and expression of antisperm antibodies in infertile couples in Kuwait", *Gynecol. Obstet. Invest.*, 45:49-53.

Pourjafari, H., Hashemzadeh Chaleshtori, M., Arab, M. (2004). "Frequencies of antigens and their allels from ABO and RH blood types in a group of women with two or more abortions", *Scientific Journal of Hamadan University of Medical Sciences*, 10:43-6.

Race, C., Ziderman, D., Watkins, W.M. (1968). "An alpha-d-galactosyltransferase associated with the blood-group B character", *Biochem. J.*, 107:733-5.

Rosenfield, R.E., Allen. F.H., Jr., Rubinstein, P. (1973). "Genetic model for the Rh blood-group system", *Proc. Natl.Acad. Sci.*, 70: 1303-1307.

Richon, J., Streiff, F., Genett, B. (1970). "Value of the Coombs-Bromeline test in ABO feto-maternal blood incompatibilities", *Bull. Fed. Soc. Gynecol. Obstet. Lang. Fr.*, 22:533-7.

Schaap, T., Shemer, R., Palti, Z. (1984). "ABO incompatibility and reproductive failure in prenatal selection", *Am. J. Hum. Genet.*, 36:143-51.

Scid Vidal J., Elies Fibla E. (2000). "Immunohematologic study of ABO hemolytic disease", *Annals. Esp. Pediatr.*, 53:249-52.

Sarici, S.U., Alpay, F., Yesilkaya, E. (2002). "Hemolytic disease of the newborn due to iso-immunization with anti-E antibodies: A case report", *Turkish J. Pediatr.*, 44:248-50.

Sharma, K., Kapoor, R. (2004). "ABO blood groups and completed reproductive performance of rural Haryanavi couples: Analysing measures of selection intensities", *J. Biosoc. Sci.*, 36:633-46.

Shen, L., Grollman, E.F., Ginsburg, V. (1968). "An enzymatic basis for secretor status and blood group substance specificity in humans", *Proc. Natl. Acad. Sci.,* USA, 59:224-30.

Soni, N., Mukherjee, B.M. (2009). "A study on foetal wastage and ABO blood groups incompatibility among the Gonds of Garriyaband, Chhattisgarh, India", *Anthropologist,* 11:229-31.

Takano, K., Miller, J.R. (1972). "ABO incompatibility as a cause of spontaneous abortion: Evidence from abortuses", *J. Med. Genet.*, 9:144-50.

Thilo, E.H., Rosenburg, A.A. (2007). "The newborn infant: Common problems in the newborn infant: Neonatal Jaundice", In: Hay, W.W., Levin, M.J., Sondheimer, J.M., (eds.) *Current Pediatric Diagnosis and Treatment,* New York: Lange Medical Books/McGraw-Hill Inc., 11-17.

Watkins, W.M., Morgan, W.T. (1959). "Possible genetical pathways for the biosynthesis of blood group mucopolysaccharides", *Vox Sang.*, 4:97-119.

Wallerstein, H. (1949). "The management of hemolytic disease of the fetus and newborn infant", *ActaHaematol.*2:349-68.

Wiene, A. (1943). "Evolution of the human blood group factors", *The American Naturalist,* 77: 199-210.

Wikman, A., Edner, A., Gryfelt, G. (2007). "Foetal hemolytic anemia and intrauterine death caused by anti-M immunization", *Transfusion,* 47:911-7.

Yoshida, A., Dave, V., Branch, D.R. *et al.* (1982). "An enzyme basis for blood type A intermediate status", *Am. J. Hum. Genet.*, 34(6):919-24.

Part-IV

Nutritional Status

12

Overweight and Socio-economic Conditions among Adult Meitei Males of Manipur

Maibam Samson Singh

Introduction

Obesity is now known to be a worldwide epidemic (Kaur *et al.*, 2008). The Department of Health, UK (2011) defined overweight and obesity as clinical terms used to describe the excess of body fat. Both overweight and obesity are often used interchangeably, but they do not represent the same situation. Some individuals may be overweight but not obese, while obese individuals are overweight above a certain degree. Obesity is a state of being seriously overweight to the stage where it becomes a risk factor for the degeneration of health. The prevalence of obesity seems to vary by sex and age across different geographical regions. Cross-sectional studies have demonstrated that obesity increases with age and that it increases most rapidly when people are in their twenties and early thirties and continues to rise until they reach their late fifties (Rolland-Cachera *et al.,* 1991; Flegal *et al.,* 1998). Prevalence of overweight and obesity has emerged across different socio-economic groups and their relationship showed inconsistent in various studies in both developed and developing countries. A consistent and strong inverse relationship has been established between economic conditions and obesity in developed countries (Albrigth *et al.,* 2005; Bove and Olson, 2006; Brodersen *et al.,* 2007; Dollman *et al.,* 2007; Mauro *et al.,* 2008). However, other investigators have reported positive relationship between economic conditions and obesity in developing countries (Reddy *et al.*, 2002; Montiero *et al.*, 2004; Fezeu *et al.*, 2006). The situation in India is more alarming, perhaps especially among the peoples of North East India among whom rural-urban migration is increasing rapidly (Khongsdier, 2008). Increasing rural-urban migration, Khongsdier (2008) continues, not only brings change in dietary and physical activity patterns but is also likely to predispose many individuals to obesity, diabetes, hypertension and other risks of CHD. The prevalence of overweight/obese among men in Sikkim, Manipur and Mizoram was 11.9 per cent, 9.2 per cent and 11.4 per cent respectively as per NFSH-2 (IIPS, 2007).

The present study has been conducted among the Meitei adults of Manipur to examine the prevalence of overweight in relation to different socio-economic conditions.

Materials and Methods

The present study was conducted among adult Meitei males residing in the urban areas of Lamphel sub-division under Imphal West District of Manipur. Imphal, the capital town of Manipur is the nodal functional centre where all the main important offices, institutions, hotels and markets are located. Different communities are living in the Imphal valley. Major portion of the population are constituted by Meitei in Imphal valley. Other communities like Muslims (Meitei Pangals) and Scheduled Caste and Scheduled Tribe population also reside in Imphal valley in small number. Cross-sectional data on 350 adult Meitei males aged between 20 and 60 years were collected following a survey of house to house visit for the present study. Data were divided as young adult (20-31 years), middle aged adult (32-45 years) and older adult (46-60 years). An anthropometric rod and a weighing scale to the nearest of 0.1 cm and 0.5 kg respectively was used to measure height and weight (Lohman *et al.*, 1998). The prevalence of overweight/obesity was calculated based on BMI following WHO International value (WHO, 2000). According to WHO classification, BMI = 30 kg/m^2 has been considered as obese and BMI between 25.0-29.9 kg/m^2, considered as overweight. BMI between 18.5-24.9 kg/m^2 indicates normal, and BMI below 18.5 kg/m^2 indicates underweight. Data on socio-economic status such as age, marital status, household income, occupation and education were collected directly from each subject using a designated schedule. Data on income was cross-checked by taking into consideration some aspects of their socio-economic condition, types of occupation, household condition and monthly expenditure. The income was divided into three categories, namely, high-income group (above 75th percentile), middle-income group (50th-75th percentile) and low-income group (below 50th percentile). Occupation was divided as government employee, business, self-employed, students and no occupation. Education was classified as secondary (class VI-X), higher secondary (class XI-XII) and graduate and above. Since the numbers of primary education adults was very negligible in number, I eventually grouped them with secondary education. The data were analysed using MS-excel and SPSS for windows, 18.0 versions. ANOVA test and chi-square test were calculated for each associated category.

Results

Table 12.1 shows the distribution of mean weight, height and BMI among adult Meitei males. Table shows that mean weight was higher among older adult (66.75±0.91) than middle aged adult (62.08±08) and young adult (60.15±0.64). The differences in mean weight were statistically significant ($p<0.01$). Mean height was more or less the same between young adult (165.24±0.51) and older adult (165.17±0.48). Mean height among middle aged adult was 164.88±0.46. The distribution of mean BMI was higher among older adult (24.44±0.30). This was higher by middle aged adult (23.79±0.26) and young adult (22.01±0.20). The differences in mean BMI in different age groups were statistically significant ($p<0.01$).

Table 12.1: Distribution of Mean Weight, Height and BMI Among Adult Meitei Males of Manipur

Age group	*N*	*Weight±SE (kg)*	*Height±SE (cm)*	*BMI±SE weight (kg)/height (m^2)*
20–31	125	60.15±0.64	165.24±0.51	22.01±0.20
32–45	104	62.08±0.83	164.88±0.46	23.79±0.26
46–60	121	66.75±0.91	165.17±0.48	24.44±0.30
Total	**350**	**63.01±048**	**165.11±0.28**	**23.08±0.15**
ANOVA Test		18.613**	0.144	24.065**

** = 0.01 level

Source: Author's Study.

Table 12.2: Prevalence of Overweight/Obesity among Adult Meitei Male of Manipur

Age group	N	Normal	Overweight/obese
20-31	125	113 (90.40%)	12 (9.60%)
32-45	106	89(83.96%)	17 (16.04%)
46-60	119	80 (67.23%)	39 (32.77%)
Total	**350**	**282 (80.57%)**	**68 (19.43%)**
		$\chi^2 = 22.029$; df = 2; p<0.001	

Source: Author's Study.

The prevalence of overweight/obesity among adult males is given in Table 12.2. Table shows that older adult males were more overweight/obesity (32.77%) followed by middle aged adult (16.04%) and young adult (9.60%). Differences in the prevalence of overweight/obesity in different age groups were significant ($\chi^2 = 22.029$; df = 2; p<0.01).

Table 12.3: Prevalence of Overweight/Obesity among Adult Meitei Male in Relation to Income

Age group	Income	N	Normal	Overweight/Obesity
20–60	HIG	95	62 (65.26%)	33 (34.74%)
	MIG	133	108 (81.20%)	25 (18.80%)
	LIG	122	112 (91.80%)	10 (8.20%)
Total		**350**	**$\chi^2 = 24.087$; df = 2, p<0.01**	

HIG = High income group; MIG = Middle income group; LIG = Low income group.

Source: Author's Study.

Prevalence of overweight/obesity with relation to income among adult Meitei males is given in Table 12.3. Table shows that adult males belong to higher income family were more overweight/obesity (34.74%). This was followed by frequency of overweight/obesity among adult males belongs to middle income family (18.80%) and lower income family (8.20%). The differences in the prevalence of overweight/obesity in different age groups were statistically significant ($\chi^2 = 24.087$; df = 2, p<0.01).

Table 12.4: Prevalence of Overweight/Obesity among Adult Meitei Males with Relation to Marital Status

Age group (year)	*Marital status*	*N*	*Normal*	*Overweight/Obesity*
20–60	Unmarried	89	79(88.76%)	10(11.24%)
	Married	261	203(77.78%)	58(22.22%)
Total		**350**	**χ^2 = 5.117, df = 1, p<0.05**	

Source: Author's Study.

Table 12.4 shows that the prevalence of overweight/obesity was higher among married males (22.22%) than the unmarried males (10.24%). The differences in different age groups were statistically significant ($\chi^2 = 5.117$, df = 1, $p<0.05$).

Table 12.5: Prevalence of Overweight/Obesity among Adult Meitei Males in Relation to Education

Age group (year)	*Education*	*N*	*Normal*	*Overweight/Obesity*
20–60	Secondary	16	12 (75.00%)	4 (25.00%)
	Hr. Secondary	117	95 (81.20%)	22 (18.80%)
	Graduate+	217	175 (80.65%)	42 (19.35%)
Total		**350**	**χ^2 = 0.347, df = 2, p>0.05**	

Source: Author's Study.

Table 12.5 shows the prevalence of overweight/obesity among adult Meitei males with relation to educational level. Prevalence of overweight/obesity (25.00%) was higher males who attained secondary level of education. The prevalence of overweight/obesity was more or less the same between adult males who attained higher secondary (18.80%) and graduate level of education (19.35%).

Table 12.6: Prevalence of Overweight/Obesity among Adult Meitei Males in Relation to Occupation

Age Group (Year)	*Occupation*	*N*	*Normal*	*Overweight/Obesity*
20–60	Govt. employee	112	69 (61.61%)	43 (38.39%)
	Business	140	121 (86.43%)	19 (13.57%)
	Self-employed	36	35 (97.22%)	1 (2.78%)
	Student	42	39 (92.86%)	3 (7.14%)
	No	20	18 (90.0%)	2 (10.00%)
Total		**350**	**χ^2 = 40.361, df = 4, p<0.01**	

Source: Author's Study.

Table 12.6 shows the prevalence of overweight/obesity among adult Meitei males with relation to occupation. Frequency of overweight/obesity (38.39%) was higher among government employees. This was followed by frequency of overweight/obesity (13.57%) among adult males who engaged in business. The prevalence of overweight/obesity among self-employed, student and no occupation was 2.78 per cent, 7.14 per cent and 10.0 per cent respectively. Prevalence of overweight/obesity among adult males in different occupational level was statistically significant ($\chi^2 = 40.361$, df = 4, $p<0.01$).

Discussion

The present study is conducted among adult Meitei males of Manipur to see the prevalence of overweight/obesity with relation to socio-economic conditions. Manipur is a small state of North East India. In the past few years, Manipur has undergone tremendous changes through rapid urbanization and socio-economic development. Such a transition has, over the years, resulted in changes among Meitei population in terms of occupation, economy, food consumption, dietary intake, physical activity levels, and overall lifestyles. Present study shows that the prevalence of overweight/obesity among Meitei adult males increases with increasing the age. Relatively lesser involvement in physical activity may be related with the higher prevalence of overweight/obesity among older people. Study shows that there is a progressive increase in the accumulation of fat in the body with increasing age (Molarious *et al.*, 2000). An increase accumulation of visceral fat in older people has been confirmed in a number of studies, and it relates to risk of diabetes and cardiovascular diseases (Goodpaster *et al.*, 2005). The positive relationship between age and obesity was also observed in earlier study (Balarajan and Villamor, 2009). Lesser involvement in exercise and the use of automobiles are certain kind of lifestyles adopted by the adult populations. Such kind of lifestyles can cause less energy expenditure from the body and increase accumulation of fat leading to the increase in body weight. The sharp increase in obesity is due to a confluence of factors, including technological advances that have lowered the costs of food, more sedentary forms of employment, and a decline in the amount of leisure time adults spend engaging in physical activity (David *et al.*, 2003).

Higher frequency of overweight/obesity among adult Meitei males belonging to the high-income families in the present study is consistent with other studies from developing countries (Monteiro *et al.*, 2004; Fezeu *et al.*, 2006). Currently, the most rapid increases in adult overweight and obesity are occurring in countries like China and India (Monteiro *et al.*, 2004). Such a rapid increase in obesity reflects the speediness of socio-economic development, nutritional transition, urbanization and modernization (Brownell, 2002; Popkin 2004). Along with the improvement of socio-economic conditions, there is also growing socio-economic differences within the populations. Such a growing differences in socio-economic conditions influence on people's dietary pattern, physical activity and over all lifestyles (Popkin and Gordon-Larson 2004; Goyal *et al.*, 2010). Rich and wealthy persons are more likely to be obese especially in developing countries as they have enough resources at their disposal to eat well and regularly (Sobal and Stunkard, 1989; Brewis, 2011). Married adult Meitei males are more overweight/ obesity in the present study is consistent with another study (Sobal *et al.*, 2009). The presence of children in a family may expose parents to snacks foods, which can lead to overweight and obesity (Sobal *et al.*, 1992). This may reflect greater parental duties and in turn less time for physical activities (Sobal *et al.,* 1992). Married individual have lower estimated daily levels of physical activities and do less physical activities in leisure time (Venters *et al.*, 1986). Prevalence of overweight/obesity is higher among adult Meitei males who attained secondary level of education. The inverse association of overweight/obesity with educational level in present study is consistent with other studies (Wardle and Griffith, 2001). However, there are also figures that show an increase in prevalence of obesity during the last decade of the twentieth century among highly educated men and women (Visscher *et al.*, 2002; Aekplakorn *et al.*, 2007). Occupational related activities coupled with relatively sedentary lifestyles could result in the increase of mean weight (Brownson *et al.*, 2005). The ever-increasing urbanization, socioeconomic improvement along with technological development, most of the occupational work can now be performed with minimum physical activities (Monda *et al.*, 2008). On the other hand, lifestyle behaviours such as motorized transportation, alcohol consumption and smoking that influence body weight are rarely considered to be related to occupation (Allman-Farinelli *et al.*, 2010). This could be reasons why government employees show the higher prevalence of overweight/obesity among adult Meitei males of Manipur.

Conclusion

The present chapter highlights the prevalence of overweight/obesity among adult Meitei males of Manipur. The prevalence of overweight/obesity increases with advancing age. Better socio-economic families are being more prone to overweight/obesity. Better socio-economic conditions may influence in dietary habits, physical activity pattern and overall lifestyles. If the increasing trend in the prevalence of overweight and obesity is not checked on time, it could lead to development of chronic morbidities associated with overweight and obesity in the adult populations. Health education programmes and effective policies are urgently required to check the increasing problems of obesity and its health consequences. Prevention should begin early in life, in childhood and adolescence. For adult, regular monitoring of BMI and fat distribution would be useful to control even modest weight gain with ageing.

References

Albright, C.L., Pruitt, L., Castro, C., Gonzalez, A., Woo, S., King, A.C. (2005). "Modifying physical activity in a multi-ethnic sample of low-income women: one-year results from the IMPACT (Increasing Motivation for Physical Activity) project", *Annals of Behav. Med.*: 30(3):191-200.

Balarajan, Y., Villamor, E. (2009). "Nationally representative surveys show recent increases in the prevalence of overweight and obesity among women of reproductive age in Bangladesh, Nepal and India", *J. Nutr.*, 139(11): 2139-2144.

Bove, C.F., Olson, C.M. (2006). "Obesity in low-income rural women: qualitative insights about physical activity and eating patterns", *Women and Health,* 44(1):57-78.

Brewis, A.A. (2011). *Obesity: Cultural and Bio-cultural Perspectives.* New Jersey: Rutgers University Press.

Brodersen, N.H., Steptoe, A., Boniface, D.R., Wardle, J. (2007). "Trends in physical activity and sedentary behaviour in adolescence: Ethnic and socio-economic differences", *Bri.T. J. Sports Med.,* 41(3):140-144.

David, M.C., Edward, L.G., Jesse, M.S. (2003). "Why have Americans become more obese?", *J. Econ. Persp.*, 17(3): 93-118.

Department of Health, UK. (2011). *Obesity General Information.* hptt://www.dh.gov.uk. Retrieved on May, 22, 2012.

Fezeu, L., Minkoulou, E., Balkau, B., Kengne, A.P., Awah, P., Unwin, N., Alberti GKMM, Mbanya, J.C. (2006). "Association between socioeconomic status and adiposity in urban Cameroon", *Int. J. Epid.*, 35(1):105-111.

Flegal, K.M., Carroll, M.D., Kuczmarski, R.J., Johnson, C.L. (1998). "Overweight and obesity in the United States: prevalence and trends", 1960-1994. *Int. J. Obes.*, 22:39-47.

Goodpaster, B.H., Krishnaswami, S., Harris, T.B., Katsiaras, A., Kritchevsky, S.B., Simonsick, E.M., Nevitt, M., Holvoet, P., Newman, A.B. (2005). "Obesity, regional body fat distribution, and the metabolic syndrome in older men and women", *Arch. Intern. Med.,* 165: 777-783.

IIPS. (2007). National Family Health Survey (NFHS-3), 2005-2006: India. Mumbai: International Institute for Population Sciences.

Kaur, S., Sachdev, H.P., Dwivedi, S.N., Lakshmy, R., Kapil, U. (2008). "Prevalence of overweight and obesity amongst school children in Delhi, India", *Asia Pac. J. Clin. Nutr.*7(4):592-596.

Khongsdier, R. (2008). "Increasing urbanization in tribal States of North East India: Implications for the prevalence of chronic diseases", *Tribes and Tribals (special Vol.).*2:25-33.

Lohman, T.G., Roch, A.F., Martorell, R. (1998). *Anthropometric Standardization Reference Manual*, Chicago: Human Kinetics Books.

Mauro, M., Taylor, V., Wharton, S., Sharma, A.M. (2008). "Barriers to obesity treatment", *Eur.J. Int. Med.*, 19:173-180.

Molarius, A., Seidell, J.C., Sans, S., Tuomilehto, J., Kuulasmaa, K. (2000). "Educational level, Relative Body Weight, and Changes in Their Association over 10 Years: An International Perspective from the WHO MONICA Project", *Am. J. Pub. Heal.,* 90:1260-1268.

Monteiro, C.A., Moura, E.C., Conde, W.L., Popkin, B.M. (2004). "Socio-economic status and obesity in adult populations of developing countries: A review", *Bull. WHO.,* 82:940-946.

Reddy, K.K.R., Rao, A.P., Reddy, T.P.K. (2002). "Socio-economic status and the prevalence of coronary heart disease risk factors", *Asia Pac. J. Clin. Nutr.,* 11(2):98-103.

Rolland-Cachera, M.F., Cole, T.J., Sempe, M., Tichet, J., Rossignol, C., Charraud, A. (1991). "Body mass index variations: centiles from birth to 87 years", *Eur. J. Clin. Nutr.*, 45:13-21.

Sobal, J., Stunkard, A.J. (1989). "Socio-economic status and obesity: A review of the literature", *Psych. Bull.,* 105:260-275.

WHO. (2000). International Association for the Study of Obesity (IASO) and International Obesity Task Force (IOTF). *The Asia-Pacific Perspective: Redefining Obesity and Its Treatment.* Geneva: World Health Organization.

13

Assessing Correlation between Socioeconomic Status and Body Mass Index

A Study of Khond of Visakhapatnam, Andhra Pradesh

Jibananda Gayen

Introduction

India is in the same queue like other highest ranking countries those are suffering from malnutrition (The World Bank Report, 2009). Apart from that, India has ranked 3rd position in South Asian Nations (SAN) immediately after Afghanistan and Pakistan and Globally 20th with a Global Hunger Index (GHI) score 29.0 (i.e. serious) (Grebmer *et al.*, 2015). Therefore, study of nutritional status among tribal community in India and their socio-economic status over the world are still relevant and augmented even in twentyfirst century since little has been done so far (Adak *et al.*, 2006; Hanson and Chen, 2006; Chakrabarty *et al.*, 2008). In India the pervasiveness of underweight children has become nearly double of countries of Sub-Saharan Africa with terrible consequences of morbidity, mortality, productivity and economic growth (Gragnolati *et al.*, 2006). Hence, undernutrition is still being noticed among the poverty-stricken people of the backward community with a few obese cases which strongly invoke some cross-sectional as well as longitudinal research activities. In the present study, tribal community especially Khond and their socio-economic statuses (SES) are considered to have an idea how socio-economic status is related with their nutrition. Nutritional statuses about this tribal group in Padmapuram village, Araku Mondal, and Andhra Pradesh are examined as it is an important aspect of health which determines a community as well as nation's future development. Thus, to measure nutritional status body mass index has been used. Body mass index is an indirect and inexpensive measure used to understand excess body weight rather than excess body fat and it is nutritionally related (WHO, 1995; Khongsdier, 2001). Body mass index (BMI) is a ratio which can be expressed as weight in kilograms to square of height in metres (kg/m^2) (Keys *et al.,* 1972). BMI solely depends upon body height and weight. It is a proxy measure of body fat because in reality, measurements of body fat takes into account the skin fold and waist circumference etc. Body mass index is an important health indicator since various levels of body mass index is correlated with body fat. However, BMI cannot be used as diagnostic tool rather it is a screening tool (Barlow and Dietz, 1998).

BMI and Health

Different health issues are related with body mass. Higher body mass index having a future health risks like cardiovascular failures, diabetes, and certain types of cancers which finally lead an individual to death (Andersen, 2003; Dishman *et al.,* 2004). Whereas, Low body mass index category sharply indicates the underweight, i.e. malnutrition which reduces immunity power and individuals are becoming more susceptible to various types of known or unknown diseases, cause of concern to public health. Malnutrition status of young children reduces their physical growth and mental development. They are becoming vulnerable in terms of their nutritional requirements. In addition to, malnutrition of pregnant women is also vulnerable because there is high propensity to give birth LBW baby which increases child morbidity and early death (Blossner and Mercedes, 2005). Malnourished girl becomes malnourished mother who otherwise maintains a cycle by providing the ballistic of malnutrition immediately to the next generation (Blossner and Mercedes, 2005).

Objectives

(*i*) To understand the nutritional status of Khond across different age and sex.

(*ii*) To know existing socio-economic status of Khond at family level.
(*iii*) To assess the correlation between socio-economic status and body mass index.
(*iv*) To assess the impact of BMI on their health.

Materials and Methods

Sampling: The sample size is determined based on the average percentage of malnutrition of Andhra Pradesh (39%). We have randomly taken 5 per cent households and 4 per cent of total tribal population of Padmapuram village as a representative sample regardless of their economic, religion and caste status.

Participants: It is a cross-sectional study conducted in Padmapuram village on Khond tribal group. Randomly 68 persons were engaged from different age groups (i.e. Girls < 20 yrs, Women >20 yrs, Boys < 20 yrs, and Men >20 yrs). A prior verbal consent was taken from the head of the family and from every individual participated. All participants belonged to Khond community.

BMI: Individual's height (mt) and weight (kg) were taken by using standard height rod and physician's balance (Model MS-02 WHITE). Each individual's body mass index (BMI) was computed [BMI = Body Weight in kg/(Body Height in m)^2]. WHO approved age and sex adjusted BMI for children and adolescents were considered and then z-score were calculated using the age and sex adjusted BMI for children and adolescents.

SES: Socio-economic status was assessed based on yearly income, capital assets (i.e. savings account, fixed deposits, LIC etc.), parents' education and occupational status of each family. Parents' occupation and education was coded using Hollingshead's Four Factor Index of Social Status (Hollingshead, 1975). Scores are given using 4 points scale. Final score of SES was calculated by standardizing and summarizing all these four factors, i.e. family income, family assets, parental occupation and parental education. High scores of SES indicate higher socio-economic status. Food habits and preferences were collected based on scheduled questionnaire. Information was also collected on communicable and non-communicable diseases they generally suffered. MS-Excel 2007 and SPSS trial version-14 software were used for data analysis.

Khond is an indigenous tribal community, inhabited in Andhra Pradesh, Odisha, Madhya Pradesh, Maharashtra, Chhattisgarh, Bihar and West Bengal (Census of India, 2011). Khond are divided into many groups according to their place of habitat, i.e. hill or *kutia* and plain dwelling Khond. Presumably, they are originated from Khondmal subdivision of Angul District, Odisha. Hence, they have the name 'Khond'. Their mother tongue is *Kui* which is very similar to Telugu. Above 92 per cent people of Padmapuram village of Araku Mandal, Andhra Pradesh district is belonging to Khond tribal group and is designated as scheduled tribes (Census of India, 2011). Initially, they are closely related with agricultural activities except few those are engaged in other forms of economic activities like business, service, construction, and handicrafts etc.

Results

Sample Characteristics Yearly family income was ranged from Rs. 24,000 to Rs. 2,40,000; 15 per cent of family had less than Rs. 24,000 annual income; 30 per cent family had less than Rs. 60,000 annual income; 25 per cent had less than Rs. 1,20,000; 20 per cent family had less than Rs. 1,80,000 annual income; 10 per cent family had greater than Rs. 2,40,000. Family assets ranged from up to Rs. 1, 00,000.

Body mass index of both girls and boys category (<20 yrs age) is unexpectedly low, i.e. 52.94 per cent girls belong to underweight (<5th percentile) and 50 per cent boys belong to underweight (<5th percentile). 47.06 per cent girls comprising healthy BMI and boys showed slightly over girls, i.e. 50 per cent.

Body mass index value for both male and female category (>20 yrs age) is not satisfactory. Slightly over 41.18 per cent female belongs to underweight (<18.5 kg) and 41.18 per cent male belongs to underweight. Female are reflecting reciprocal picture in adult age group which is 52.94 per cent in healthy BMI level. Male are equal sharing, i.e. 41.18 per cent both in underweight and healthy BMI category. Male has 5.88 per cent obese tendency but female has no obese tendency but showing little bit overweight status, i.e. 5.88 per cent which is also slightly high in male counterpart, i.e. 11.76 per cent (Figs. 13.1 to 13.4).

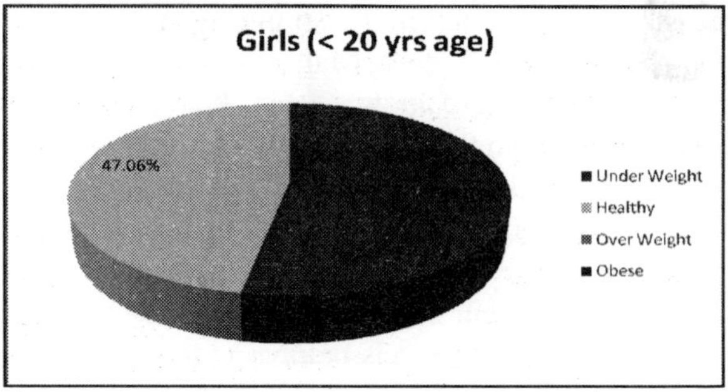

Fig. 13.1: BMI of Girls (<20 yrs age)

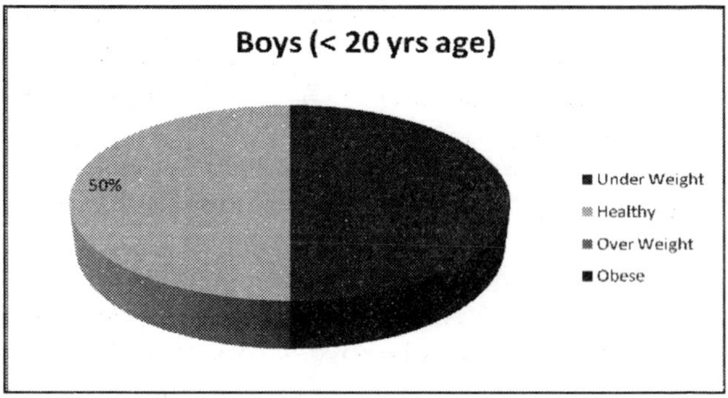

Fig. 13.2: BMI of Boys (<20 yrs age)

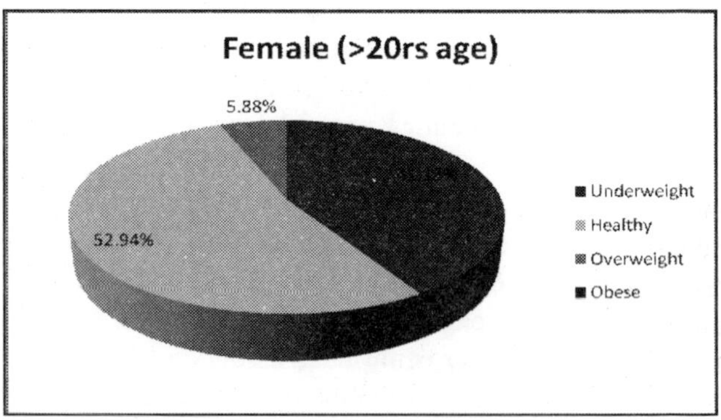

Fig. 13.3: BMI of Male (>20 yrs age)

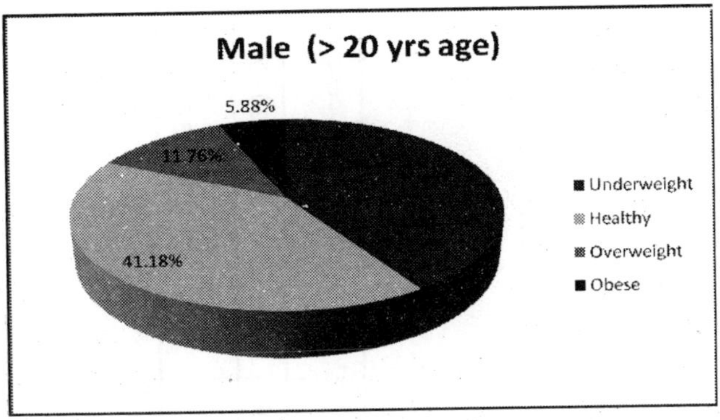

Fig. 13.4: BMI of Female (>20 yrs age)

Boys (< 20 yrs age) have mean BMI value 15.402 and Z-score varies between-1.141 to 2.296. Girls (< 20 yrs age) have mean BMI value 14.936 and Z-score varies between –1.15 to 1.721. Male (>20 yrs age) have mean BMI value 20.327 and Z-score varies between 1.642 and 2.318. Female (>20 yrs age) have mean BMI value 19.879 and Z-score varies between 1.416 and 1.707 (Table 1). Importantly, Girls and Female both have low BMI.

The obtained BMI values of above 20 yrs age were also tallied and classified on the basis of chronic energy deficiency (CED) grades (James *et al.,* 1988; Ferro-Luzzi *et al.,* 1992; WHO, 1995). 41.17 per cent female suffers by chronic energy deficiency (CED). But, females have no overweight or obese tendency which augments their social position as well. Only 29.41 per cent males reflect normal condition whereas 47.06 per cent are suffering from chronic energy deficiency. Only 17.65 has overweight tendency and 5.88 per cent males (Table 13.2) has obese tendency which clearly establishes higher nutrition shares contrary to women even in tribal community.

Above 90 per cent people are suffering from fever. A certain amount of people suffered from skin disease, diarrhoea, dysentery and cold and cough because of the poor environmental conditions as well as low immunity due to malnutrition. Other diseases include headache, body pain, and arthritis having some linkages with food preferences and malnutrition.

Discussion

It has been observed that BMI among tribal community especially

Table 13.1: Mean and SD Value of Age, Height, Weight and BM and Z Scores

Sex	Age (Yrs)		Height (m)		Weight (kg)		BMI		Z Score	
	Mean (x)	SD (σ)	Mean (x)	SD (σ)	Mean (x)	SD (σ)	Mean (x)	SD (σ)	Min	Max
Boys (<20yrs Age)	10.441	5.011	131.176	22.950	27.823	13.682	15.402	3.138	–1.141	2.296
Girls (<20yrs Age)	8.631	5.286	119.210	30.491	24	13.871	14.936	2.580	–1.500	1.721
Male (>20yrs Age)	46.647	14.684	154.411	6.996	48.823	13.669	20.327	5.076	–1.642	2.318
Female (>20yrs Age)	33.588	11.807	150	7.071	44.764	7.573	19.879	2.864	–1.416	1.707

Source: Author's Study.

Table 13.2: Chronic Energy Deficiency Status

Sex	CED STATUS					
	CED grade III (severe thinness)	CED grade II (moderate thinness)	CED grade I (mild thinness)	Normal	Overweight	Obese
	< 16.00	16.00-16.99	17.00-18.49	18.50-24.99	25.00-29.99	?30.00
Female >20 yrs	5.88 %	11.76 %	23.53 %	58.82 %	–	–
Male >20 yrs	17.65 %	11.76 %	17.65 %	29.41 %	17.65 %	5.88 %

Source: Author's Study.

Khond is significantly low. Moreover, SES of the tribal group is also significantly associated with their Body Mass Index (BMI). Proportional relationship between socio-economic status and BMI has been identified among Khond. Boys and girls who are under age (< 20 yrs age) having low SES have lower BMI. Men and women who are aged (< 20 yrs age) having low SES had lower BMI. On the other level, BMI and weight is significantly associated with SES. Weight is also statistically significant with age of people. Since, weight is waning with increasing age is reflected in this study. This research has specifical two findings. First, is in our tests BMI of Khond is highly correlated with SES (r = 0.776). Instead of other factors impacted on BMI a single factor, here, is highly significant. Secondly, average BMI of tribal community especially Khond, is unexpectedly low in Padmapuram Village. It is emerged from our research that people from lower socio-economic background had low BMI because they are incapable to access nutritious food, medical facilities, hence, are more susceptible to different types of communicable and non-communicable diseases some of which are of unknown origin.

BMI is proportionally correlated with their socio-economic status. Value of r is 0.776 which suggests very strong correlation exists. R^2 = 0.603 which clearly shows strong relation between BMI and SES (Fig. 13.6). Weight and BMI is also highly correlated (r = 0.909). SES has some amount of positive impact on weight (r = 0.695) (Table 13.3).

Understanding the nutritional status of a community through BMI will address status of public health which promotes priority based planning to eradicate such societal disparities. It has been observed that there is an inseparable relation between physical illness and nutritional status of any community in addition to other factors include literacy percentage, work participation rate of both male and female, per capita income, purchasing power, and way of living etc. Reasons of different illness and their relation with nutrition will help us to curb undernutrition by providing Study some welfare centric central projects. This work initially highlighted that gaps in health in a quantitative way (Figs. 13.1 to 13.4) and also showed how people are suffering from different physical illness due to lack of optimum nutrition (Fig. 13.5). Therefore, this cross-sectional study would surely benefit with their findings in the public health arena.

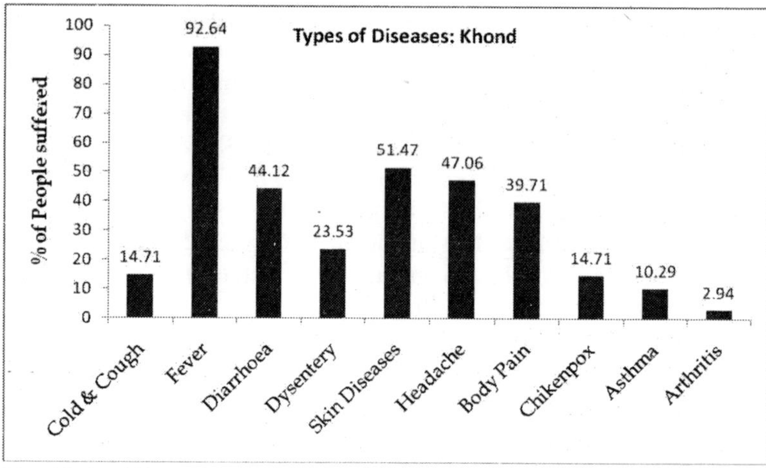

Fig. 13.5: Different physical ailments

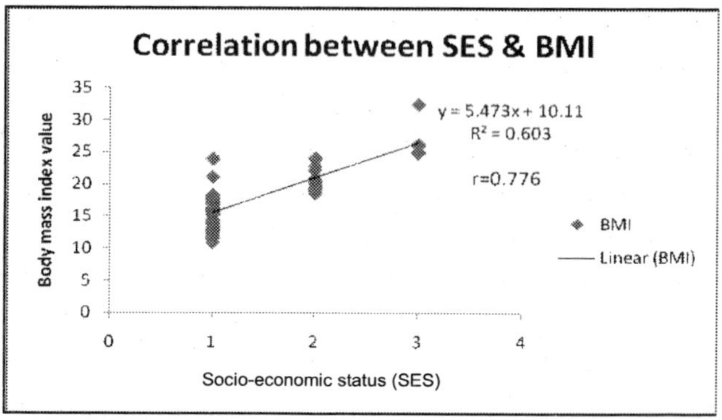

Fig. 13.6: Correlation between BMI and SES

Conclusion

Literacy rate of Khond is 59 per cent which is quite low in respect of National literacy rate, i.e. 73 per cent. Nutritional status among Khond is breath taking. Fifty one per cent of adolescents having age < 20 yrs belong to underweight status and slightly over 41 per cent adults having age >20 yrs belong to underweight category. GDP per capita income of India is US$ 1861.50 whereas 45 per cent people have the annual income less than Rs. 60,000. In spite of the ample numbers of central backward welfare projects are already implemented the scenario of tribal life is not healthy yet which not only bring intolerable

Table 13.3: Correlation Matrix Showing Nature of Association

	SES	*BMI*	*Weight (kg)*	*Height (m)*	*Age*	*Gender*
SES	1					
BMI	0.776	1				
Weight (kg)	0.695	0.909	1			
Height (m)	0.138	0.162	0.104	1		
Age	0.288	0.470	–0.597	–0.044	1	
Gender	–0.072	–0.081	–0.129	–0.123	–0.065	1

Source: Author's Study.

miseries to their life rather quite unexpected even in second decade of twenty first century. Village-wise door to door survey is necessary to unravel the real information and policy measures to be taken, priority basis to understand, framing and solving the problems of time immemorial.

Acknowledgements

The author deeply acknowledges the role of Khond people of Padmapuram Village who not only have participated in the interviewing schedule, but they had shared their socio-economic information, food habit and preferences, information on different types of diseases they suffered and helping in anthropometric measurements. The author is thankful to his beloved B.Sc. final year students of 2015 and his colleague, Mrs. Srimayi Biswas, for her worthy contribution with data collection.

References

Adak, D.K., Gautam, R.K. and Gharami, A.K. (2006). "Assessment of nutritional status through body mass index among adult males of 7 tribal populations of Maharashtra, India", *Malaysian Journal of Nutrition, 12*(1), 23-31.

Andersen, R. (2003). *Obesity: Etiology, Assessment, Treatment, and Prevention. Human Kinetics.*

Barlow, S.E. and Dietz, W.H. (1998). "Obesity evaluation and treatment: Expert committee recommendations", *Pediatrics, 102*(3), e29-e29.

Blössner, M., De Onis, M., and Prüss-Üstün, A. (2005). *Malnutrition: Quantifying the Health Impact at National and Local Levels*. Geneva: World Health Organization.

Delhi, N. (2011). Office of the Registrar General and Census Commissioner, Ministry of Home Affairs, Government of India; 2014. *Population Projections for India and States.*

Chakrabarty, S., Pal, M., Bharati, S. and Bharati, P. (2008). "Body form and nutritional status among adult males of different social groups in Orissa and Bihar States in India". *HOMO-Journal of Comparative Human Biology, 59*(3):235-251.

Dishman, R., Heath, G. and Lee, I.M. (2012). *Physical Activity Epidemiology,* 2nd edition. Human Kinetics.

Ferro-Luzzi, A., Sette, S., Franklin, M., and James, W.P. (1992). "A simplified approach of assessing adult chronic energy deficiency". *European Journal of Clinical Nutrition, 46*(3): 173-186.

Gragnolati, M., Shekar, M., Dasgupta, M., Bredenkamp, C. and Lee, Y.K. (2016). India's undernourished children: a call for reform and action. Health, Nutrition and Population (HNP) discussion paper. World Bank.

Grebmer, K.V., Bernstein, J., Prasai, N., Yin, S., Yohannes, Y. and Waal, A.D. (2015). *Global Hunger Index: Armed Conflict and the Challenge of Hunger-2015.* International Food Policy Research Institute.

Hanson, M.D. and Chen, E. (2006). "Socio-economic status, race, and body mass index: The mediating role of physical activity and sedentary behaviours during adolescence", *Journal of Pediatric Psychology, 32*(3): 250-259.

Hollingshead, A.B. (1975). *Four Factor Index of Social Status*, New Haven, CT.

James, W.P.T., Ferro-Luzzi, A. and Waterlow, J.C. (1988). "Definition of chronic energy deficiency in adults". *Eur. J. Clin. Nutr.*, 42: 969-981.

Keys, A., Fidanza, F., Karvonen, M.J., Kimura, N., and Taylor, H.L. (1972). "Indices of relative weight and obesity". *Journal of Chronic Diseases, 25*(6-7): 329-343.

Khongsdier, R. (2001). "Body mass index of adult males in 12 populations of Northeast India". *Annals of Human Biology, 28*(4): 374-383.

World Bank (2009). Retrieved 2009-07-17. *World Bank Report on Malnutrition in India.*

World Health Organization (WHO) (1995). Physical status. The use and interpretation of anthropometry. *WHO Technical Report No. 854*. WHO, Geneva.

14

Nutrition Status of the Hand Rickshaw Pullers of Kolkata

A Case Study

Pranab Kr. Das

Introduction

In present day India, we find that the most feudal systems are surviving at the heart of modern cities. Metropolitan Kolkata's informal sector is the prime destination for those who cannot obtain jobs in the formal sectors. Informal sectors employ more than 40 per cent of the total labour force of the Kolkata (Chakravorty, 2000). Migration and urbanisation are the integral parts of economic development and social transformation. They are the barometers of changing socio-economic and political conditions at the national and international levels (Deshingkar and Aktar, 2009). Hand pulled rickshaw of Kolkata is one of such feudal-colonial system which provides job to the marginalised migrant people from Bihar, Jharkhand (Mitra, 1982). However, a considerable number of Bengalis are also engaged in this occupation, they are mostly from neighbouring districts of Kolkata. Rickshaw pulling is an extraordinary physical effort with high caloric needs like the athletes (Banerjee, 1959). Nutrition and health both have great influence in labour market, basically in unorganised sectors. As a component of human capital, health is a key factor in the creation of wealth (Mwabu, 1998). Lucas (1993) emphasises productivity growth as the source of economic miracles in East Asian countries. In the Indian context, Gupta and Mitra (2003) found a positive relationship between economic growth and health. Studies in the recent past in India show a strong negative association of income/consumption expenditure to morbidity (Duraisamy, 1998) implying less morbidity leading to higher living status. With the advent of efficiency wage hypothesis and its nutrition-based variant (Leibenstein, 1957), this question has been addressed very much in contemporary development studies. In this context, the present study explores the nutrition and health status of the hand rickshaw pullers of Kolkata highlighting their socio-economic condition.

There are several techniques to measure nutrition level and health status. Weight for height (wasting) and height for age (stunting) are two widely accepted indicators to understand the nutritional status of an individual, especially children (Fogel, 1997, Thomas and Strauss, 1997). In case of adults, the most widely accepted measures are Body Mass Index. BMI is related to energy intake, net of output; it has also been shown to be related to maximum oxygen uptake during physical work, which is, in turn, related to aerobic capacity and endurance, independent of energy intake (Spurr, 1983; Martorell and Arroyave, 1988). Hence, for the jobs that require sustained physical effort, this is an important pathway through which health may influence worker's productivity. Moreover, energy can be stored in the body and expended when needed, which implies that BMI may be affected by contemporaneous movements in incomes or prices, so that the dynamics linking BMI and productivity may be very complicated. Persistence of positive correlation between wages and BMI for those with a very low or zero level of education indicates that among men with no education, BMI plausibly is associated with greater physical strength, which is of value for manual labour (Strauss and Thomas, 1998). It is found that BMI, which is a good proxy for current health and nutritional status of adults, is highly correlated with adult mortality rates (Fogel, 1994). BMI, which tends to be subject to diminishing returns (Thomas and Strauss, 1997), is also approximately orthogonal to height; therefore, both may be included as determinants of productivity without introducing severe multicollinearity among regressors (Schultz, 2005). However, BMI varies with ethnicity, topology, and climate; so it is not very useful in comparing the nutritional status of the different group of individuals. A very new and different type of technique to assess the adult nutrition level is daily caloric expenditure against daily caloric intake in respect of physical activity factor, RMR, TEE and TEF (Manini, 2010 & Edward,

2013). In recent past, few techniques have been developed to measure nutritional levels which are based on food image processing through Support Vector Machine Algorithm. This system takes the images of food and using image processing and segmentation, it calculates the nutrition and calorie content in the food (Podutwar, 2016). Another technique has been developed based on android technology. Where an android application is used to track the user physical activity and estimate his or her energy expenditure using 3 axis accelerometer and GPS in a Smartphone with an android operating system (Pal and Hepsiba, 2013). However, last two methods are still not so popular in public domain.

The main objective of this intensive case study is to explore the nutrition status of the hand rickshaw pullers of Kolkata. This chapter also explores the daily caloric intake and expenditure of the hand rickshaw pullers with specific formula and methods. Moreover, it discusses the common health disorders of the rickshaw pullers which are associated with the malnutrition.

Methodology

The daily caloric intake and expenditure of the hand rickshaw pullers are specially calculated in this study. For the calculation of Daily Caloric Expenditure, the FAO & WHO Expert Consultation method is used which is also suggested by T.M. Manini in 2010 and Edward in 2013. For the Daily Caloric Intake, the calorie value of different food items is considered with various dietary combinations consumed by both Bengali and Non-Bengali rickshaw pullers. ICMR standard is considered to measure caloric value of the individual food which is also used by the fitness website Appololife.

Calculation of Daily Caloric Intake

To understand the food habit and dietary combination of the rickshaw pullers, 250 were surveyed through purposive random sampling from different pockets of Kolkata city. From the field survey and personal observation, it is noticed that rice is the staple food for the Bengali rickshaw pullers and *chapatti* for non-Bengalis. However, most of non-Bengalis are taking rice in lunch. It is simply because most of them (non-Bengalis) usually have their lunch in *pice* hotels, which provide rice at a low rate and in dinner they prepare *chapattis* in group mess. So, dietary choices for both are different. At lunch and afternoon snacks, they eat at same places, so there is no such variation in dietary combination. But, in breakfast and dinner, they prefer their traditional food and so that there are variations in food preferences. From the interviews and personal observations, these dietary components or elements are found, consumed by the rickshaw pullers, listed in Table 14.1 with calorie values. The dietary combinations of breakfast, lunch, afternoon snacks and dinner are accordingly given in table format from Tables 14.2 to 14.5 with calorie value and daily average calorie intakes of hand rickshaw pullers are shown in Table 14.6. So, average calorie intake of the hand rickshaw pullers is 3884.35 cal/day/person.

Table 14.1: Calorie Value of Consumed Dietary Components of Hand Rickshaw Pullers

Food Items	*Amount*	*Food Value in Calories*
Rice (Boiled)	100 gm	216*
Chapatti	100 gm	286*
Sattu	100gm	400*
Mixed Vegetables	100 gm	75*
Dal (Bengal gram)	100 gm	119*
Full egg	1 piece	78*
Fish Deep Fry	100 gm	112*
Paneer	100 gm	357*
Chicken Curry	100 gm	190*
Milk	100 ml	100*
Tea with milk and Sugar	1 cup	151*
Puffed Rice	100 gm	402*
Chop or *Pakora* (potato)	3 piece	280*
Butter and Bread	4 piece	360*
Channa	100 gm	269*

*as per Appololife based on ICMR standard.
Source: Fieldwork.

Table 14.2: Dietary Combinations for Breakfast.

Preferable diet for Bengali HRP	*Calorie value*	*Preferable diet for Non-Bengali HRP*	*Calorie value*	
Tea One Cup	151	Tea One Cup	151	
Chapatti 4 (200 gm) and vegetables	602 +59	*Sattu* 200 gm	800	
Total	**812**	**Total**	**951**	**χ^2 881.50**

Source: Fieldwork.

Table 14.3: Dietary Combinations for Lunch

Common Food items with amount (Average estimation)	*Calorie value*	*Variable items in menu with amount (Average estimation)*	*Calorie Value*	*Food Combination*	*Calorie Value*
Rice 350 gm	756.00	Egg 1 piece	78.00	Rice+ mixed vegetables +Dal	954.00
Mixed Vegetable Curry (200 gm)	150.00	Egg 2 pieces	156.00	Rice+ mixed vegetables +Dal + one egg	1032.00
Bengal gram *Dal* (40gm)	48.00	Fish 100 gm	112.00	Rice+ mixed vegetables +Dal+ two egg	1110.00
		Paneer 150 gm	357.00	Rice+ mixed vegetables +Dal +Fish	1066.00
		Chicken 200 gm	380.00	Rice+ mixed vegetables +Dal + paneer	1311.00
				Rice+ mixed vegetables +Dal +Chicken	1334.00

Source: Fieldwork.

Table 14.4: Dietary Combinations of Afternoon Snacks

Common Item	*Calorie Value*	*Variable items with quantity or amount*	*Caloric Value*	*Combination*	*Caloric Value*
Tea (one Cup)	151	Puffed rice (50 gm)	201	One cup tea + Puffed Rice + Chops	632.00
		Chops/Pakora (3 piece)	280		
				One cup tea + Puffed Rice + Channa	621.00
		Bread butter (4 piece)	360		
				One cup tea + Bread Butter	511.00
		Double Egg Omelet	156		
				One cup tea + Double Egg Omelet+ Puffed rice	508.00
		Channa (100 gm)	269		
				One cup tea + Channa + Double omelet	576.00
					χ^2 **569.60**

Source: Fieldwork.

Table 14.5: Dietary Combinations for Dinner

Preferable Dietary items of Non Bengali HRP with amount	*Calorie Value*	*Preferable Dietary items of Bengali HRP with amount*	*Calorie Value*	*Food Combination*	*Total Calorie Value*
Chapatti (6 piece or 350 gm)	1001	Rice 350 gm	756.00	Rice + mixed vegetables + Dal + Milk (250 ml)	1204.00
Mixed Vegetable Curry (250 gm)	187.5	Mix Vegetable Curry (200 gm)	150.00	Rice + mixed vegetables + Dal + one egg	1032.00
		Bengal gram Dal (40 gm)	48.00	Rice + mixed vegetables + Dal + Fish	1066
Full Cream Milk (250 ml)	250.00	Fish 100 gm	112	Rice + mixed vegetables + Dal + Chicken	1334
		Egg 1 piece	78.00		
		Chicken 200 gm	380		
Total Caloric Value 1438.50 cal		**(1438.50 + 1159/2) cal = 1298.75cal**		**χ^2 1159 cal**	

Source: Fieldwork.

Table 14.6: Daily Average Calorie Intakes of Hand Rickshaw Pullers

Intake period	*Dietary intake value in cal/day*
Break Fast	881.50
Lunch	1134.50
Afternoon Snacks	569.60
Dinner	1298.75
Total	**3884.35 Cal/day**

Source: Fieldwork.

Calculation of Daily Caloric Expenditures

For the calculation of daily caloric expenditures, three terms are needed to be understood; *Resting Metabolic Rate* (RMR), *Thermal Effect of Exercise* (TEE) and *Thermal Effect of Food* (TEF).

Resting Metabolic Rate: Resting metabolic rate (RMR) is the energy that has been spent while at rest (expressed in calorie/day). However, the actual value of RMR depends on age, sex, body weight etc. Table 14.7 provides the RMR for male.

Table 14.7: Estimating RMR for Male

Age Range in Years	*Equation for RMR (Calories/Day)*
0–3	(60.9 × weight) – 54
3–10	(22.7 × weight) + 495
11–18	(17.5 × weight) + 651
19–30	(15.3 × weight) + 679
31–60	(11.6 × weight) + 879
>60	(13.5 × weight) + 487

Source: FAO/WHO Expert Consultation Method.

Thermal Effect of Exercise: The term Thermal Effect of Exercise means, the energy spent due to activity over and above RMR (FAO/WHO Expert Consultation, 2001). Actually TEE depends on the activity of a person.

Equation for TEE = RMR ×Activity Factor

There are four levels of activities such as Sedentary, Lightly Active, Moderately Active, Very Active, and Extremely Active (Edward, 2013) which are shown in Table 14.8.

Thermic Effect of Food: It is the amount of energy expenditure above the RMR due to the cost of processing food for use and storage (Edward, 2013). Actually, it is that energy which is used in digestion,

Table 14.8: Level of Activity and Activity Factors

Level of Activities	*Example*	*Activity Factors*
Sedentary	Office worker getting little or no exercise	1.40–1.69
Moderately Active	Construction worker, Truck Driver, Postal Peon etc.	1.70–1.99
Very Active	Full time athletes, unskilled labourers, some agricultural workers (especially peasant farming), forestry workers, army recruits and soldiers in active service, mine workers, steel workers.	2.00–240
Extremely Active	Lumberjacks, blacksmiths, female construction workers, heavy manual digging, **rickshaw pullers**, and coal mining. Moderate to high level of physical activity for most of the work day or exercise comparable to running 14 to 17 miles/day.	>2.40

Source: FAO/WHO Expert Consultation Method.

absorption and distribution of nutrients. However, TET can be varied for different dietary elements, but commonly it is estimated that TET is 10 per cent of calorie intake of a person.

To apply this formula, ten rickshaw pullers were randomly selected from different parts of the city belongs to different age groups, religions, castes. The result is found as in Table 14.9. One example is illustrating for understanding the calculation steps.

Name of Hand Rickshaw Puller: Md. Anwar, Age: 45, Sex: Male, Weight: 62

Step 1: Calculation for Resting Metabolic Rate (RMR)

Formula for calculating RMR = 11.6 × (weight) + 879 (for age group of 31–60 years)

$$11.6 \times 62 + 879 = 1598.2 \text{ calories/day}$$

Step 2: Calculations for Thermal Effect of Exercise (TEE)

Formula for TEE = RMR ×Activity Factor
1598.2 × 2.4 (As shown in Table 14.8)
= 3835.68 calories/day

Step 3: Calculations for Estimated Daily Calorie Expenditure (EDCE)

Formula for EDCE = TEE + Thermic Effect of Food (TEF) i.e. 10 per cent of TEE
3835.68 Calories + 383.56 Calories
= 4219.24 Calories/Day
or 4219 Calories/Day

So, Md. Anwar's daily minimum estimated calorie expenditure is 4219.

Similarly, estimated calorie expenditure of ten selected hand rickshaw pullers is shown in Table 14.9 as per FAO/WHO Expert Consultation parameter and formula.

So, as per Table 14.9 the average estimated daily caloric expenditure of the hand rickshaw pullers is 4005 calorie.

Table 14.9: Minimum Estimated Calorie Expenditure of Ten Selected Hand Rickshaw Pullers of Kolkata as per FAO/WHO Expert Consultation Parameter and Formula

Name	*Sex*	*Location of Stands*	*Age in Years*	*Weight*	*Equation for RMR (Calories/Day)*	*Activity factors*	*TEE (RMR × Activity factor)*	*Thermic Effect of Food (10% of TEE)*	*Estimated Daily Calorie Expenditure (TEE + 10% of TEE)*
Md. Anwar	M	11 C R. G Kar Road (Shyam Bazar), Kol-04	45	62.00	(11.6 × weight) + 879 = 1598.2	2.4	3835.68	383.56	4219
Surya Yadav	M	74/6 A Bagbazar (Near Post Office), Kol-03	18	61.00	(17.5 × weight) + 651 = 1718.50		4124.4	412.44	4537
Bhusan Sharma	M	Cornfield Road, Kol-19 (Ballygunj)	65	57.50	(13.5 × weight) + 487 = 1263.25		3031.8	303.18	3334
Kali Das	M	Sealdah (Near South Station), Kol-14	30	55.00	(15.3 × weight) + 679 = 1520.5		3649.2	364.92	4014
Sheak Nawsar	M	A.P.C. Road (Near Victoria College), Kol-9	45	59.80	(11.6 × weight) + 879 = 1572.68		3774.43	377.44	4152
Sanju Maahaldar	M	Lake Market, Rashbehari Avenue, Kol-26	25	65.00	(15.3 × weight) + 679 = 1673.5		4016.4	401.64	4418
Nirdhan Paswan	M	Kalighat Temple Road, Kali Temple, Kol-26	55	68.60	(11.6 × weight) + 879 = 1674.76		4019.42	401.94	4421
Degan Yadav	M	College Street, Bata Junction, Kol-9	45	57.00	(11.6 × weight) + 879 = 1540.2		3686.48	368.64	4065
Tulsi Prasad	M	M.G. Road (Near Surendra Nath College, Kol-9	65	53.50	13.5 × (weight) + 487 = 1209.25		2902.2	290.22	3192
Harak Palhad Ram	M	114, Princep Street (Near Hanuman Temple), Kol-72	45	63.00	(11.6 × weight) + 879 = 1401		3362.4	336.24	3699
									χ^2 **4005** SD = 436.185

Source: FAO/WHO Expert Consultation Method.

Results

Average Daily Calorie Intake of hand rickshaw pullers is 3884.35 Cal/day (Table 14.6) which is lower than their average daily Estimated Calorie Expenditure (ECE), i.e. 4005 as per WHO, FAO Expert Consultation Method (Table 14.9). The hand rickshaw pullers are taking a lesser amount of food than their requirements. Pulling rickshaw is an extreme effort, more laborious than professional athletes. These persons averagely run more than 25 km per day to operate their business in extremely harsh conditions. They usually burn more calorie than their intake, so, the majority of them are suffering from malnutrition and related health disorders.

To understand the relation between nutrition and health, 250 surveyed hand rickshaw pullers were specially asked about their common health problems, suffering since last two years. Among the surveyed rickshaw pullers 65.6 per cent informed positively that they have some common physical problems and rest 35.4 per cent responded negatively. Rickshaw pullers mainly complained about fatigue (26.83%) followed by the breathing problem, back pain, headache, musculoskeletal pain and heart palpitation (Fig. 14.1). All these health disorders are very much associated with the low-calorie intake and poor level of nutrition.

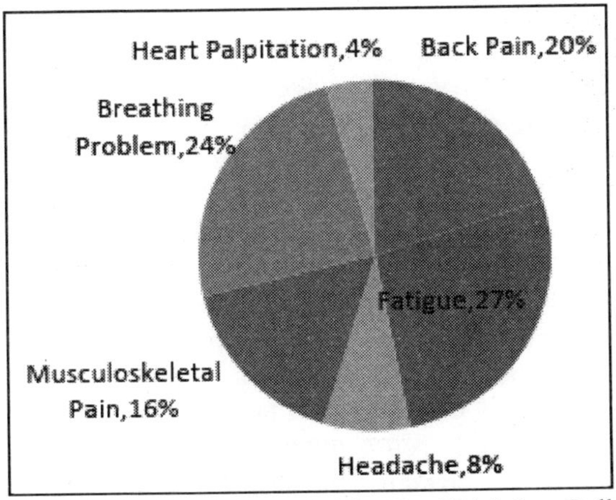

Fig. 14.1: Common Physical Problems of the Hand Rickshaw Pullers.

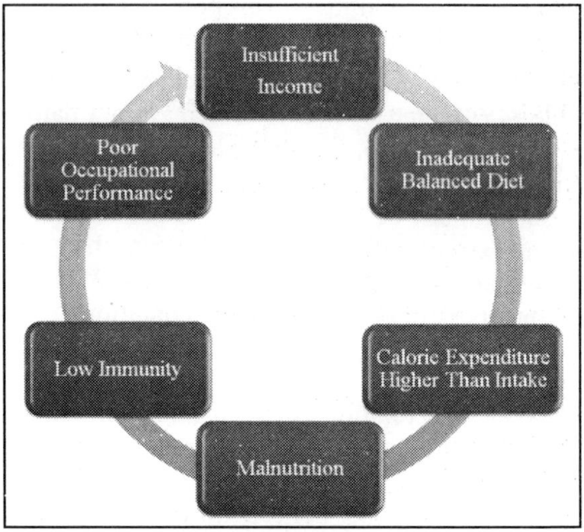

Fig. 14.2: Relationship among the Nutrition Level, Health Status, Occupational Performance and Income.

Discussions

We produce energy from metabolism after having food. Calories are found from the biological molecules of food that we eat. After burning these biological molecules through cellular respiration we release this energy for energy-requiring processes such as normal metabolism and physical activity. When we eat more calories than our requirements, the excess calories may be stored as glycogen, fat, cholesterol etc. in our tissues and organs. Consequently, we gain weight. If we burn more calories than we eat, stored biological molecules in our tissues and organs must be used to meet these expenditures and we begin to lose weight. So, it is clear that maintaining a healthy body weight is really just a matter of balancing caloric intake and expenditure. There is a positive correlation between income and caloric intake. It is observed that poor people generally take less amount of food than the persons having stable financial condition. Stable and secure income guarantees food supply and consumption to any person. But the hand rickshaw pullers are in extreme poverty facing challenges and difficulties in a cosmopolitan atmosphere without proper knowledge and skills. They expense minimum for food to ensure good remittances for families. Average daily income of the rickshaw pullers is only Rs. 210.74 (as per primary survey) including all expenditures. This poor income is not sufficient to ensure adequate diet for them, so their daily caloric expenditure is higher than intake and they are suffering from malnutrition which hampers their health, occupational performance and income (Fig. 14.2). The hand rickshaw pullers of Kolkata are the perfect example of poverty cycle.

This intensive case study is helpful to understand the nutrition and health status of the hand rickshaw pullers of Kolkata. In future, there is further scope to increase the volume of the data for more authentic and relevant results. The methodology of the present studies is very much contemporary and useful for the research related to the public health issue, mainly for unskilled labourers. In these studies, nutrition level of the hand rickshaw pullers is measured through FAO & WHO Expert Consultation method and formula which based on daily caloric intake, expenditure and activity factors. This method could be used for other occupational groups as per their types of work and activity factors.

Conclusion

Generally, health of an individual person mostly depends on his or her nutrition level. Nutritious food is very important for substantial physical and mental development. Nutrition level and health status both are closely related to the quality of life. Better quality of life ensures long life expectancy. In India, the nutrition level and health condition of a person or social group is very much associated with socio-economic status; which includes income, education, family status and work conditions. Occupational performances, income and job security are very much depended on to health status. There is a positive correlation in nutrition level and economic condition. Food security is an important matter in the contemporary world. Malnutrition, hunger, morbidity etc. are the chronic problems in the developing countries. In Kolkata, hand rickshaw-pullers are such labourers, bearing colonial heritage with maximum tolerance and ignorance. They are in the extreme poverty and living life a little better than the beggars. They are taking food only to live. They have to send remittances on a regular basis. So, they spend a minimum on food and they are mostly suffering from malnutrition and associated health disorders. It is observed that their carbohydrate intake is higher than protein and fat due to poor income. Moreover, their health condition becomes more critical due to lack of knowledge in health and hygiene. Here it is important to say that one hand rickshaw puller runs more than 25 km per day with the load factor so their activity factor should be higher than 2.40 (activity factor of extremity activity section). So, the actual Estimated Caloric Expenditure (ECE) would be higher than Table 14.9, this table shows the minimum ECE of the pullers. They usually burn more calorie than their intake and they are very much underweight. The majority of the rickshaw pullers are very slim, always tired, looked more aged than their actual age and facing low immunity. So, they are very much vulnerable to life-threatening infectious diseases such as influenza, typhoid, tuberculosis, hepatitis, jaundice, amoebiasis, diarrhoeal diseases and skin infection including vector born diseases.

References

Banerjee, S., Acharya, N.K. and Chattopadhyay, D.P. (1959). "Studies on energy expenditure of rickshaw pullers, Calcutta", *Indian Journal of Philology*, 6, pp. 147-160.

Chakravorty, S. (2000). "From colonial city to global city: The far from complete spatial transformation of Calcutta," In: Peter Marcuse and Roland van Kempen (eds.) *Globalization Cities: A New Spatial Order*? Oxford: Blackwell Publishing, p. 72.

Deshingkar, P. and Akter, S. (2009). *Migration and Human Development in India, Human Development, UNDP Human Development Reports Research Paper 2009/13*, UNDP, London, p. 102.

Duraisamy, P. (2001). "Health status and curative health care in rural India", *Working Paper Series No.78*, National Council of Applied Economic Research, New Delhi, pp. 12-38.

Fogel, R. (1994). "Economic growth, population theory, and physiology: The bearing of long-term processes on the making of economic policy", *American Economic Review*, 84: 369-395.

Germano, Mwabu (1998). Health Development in Africa, *Economic Research Papers No. 38*. African Development Bank, pp. 42-60.

Goljan, Edward F. (2013). "Rapid review pathology", *Health Sciences*, Elsevier, Oklahoma, p. 174.

Gupta, Indrani and Mitra, A. (2003). "Economic growth, health and poverty: An exploratory study on India", In: Mishra, P., R. Chatterjee, and S. Rao (eds), *India Health Report*, New Delhi: Oxford University Press, p. 122.

"Human energy requirements: Energy Requirement of Adults", *Report of a Joint FAO/WHO Expert Consultation*, Rome: Food and Agriculture Organization of the United Nations, available online: http://www.fao.org/docrep/007/y5686e/y5686e00.htm (accessed on 18 April 2016).

Leibenstein, Harvey (1957). "The theory of underemployment in backward economies", *The Journal of Political Economy*, 65(2): 91-103.

Lucas, Robert E. (1988). "On mechanics of economic development", *Journal of Monetary Economics*, 22(1):3 42.

Manini, T.M. (2010). "Energy expenditure and aging", *Ageing Research Reviews*, 9 (1): pp. 1-11.

Martorell, R. and G. Arroyave (1988). "Malnutrition, work output and energy laceds", In: Collins, K. and Roberts F. (eds.), *Capacity for Work in the Tropics*. Cambridge: Cambridge University Press, pp. 52-59.

Mitra, Asim (1982). *The Rickshaw Wallas and the Thella Wallas in Calcutta: Aspects of Society and Culture in Calcutta,* Calcutta: Anthropological Survey of India, p. 199.

Pal, Bhabani Sankar, Hepsiba, D. (2013), "Real time monitoring of daily calorie expenditure using smart phone", *International Journal of Advanced Research In Computer Science and Software Engineering,* 3(3):268-273.

Podutwar, A.A., Shinde, A.V. (2016). "Calorie and nutrition measurement based on food image processing", *International Journal of Recent Trends in Engineering and Research (IJRTER),* 2(4): 253-256.

Schultz, T.P., 1998, "The formation of human capital and the economic development of Africa: Returns to health and schooling investments", *Economic Research Papers* No. 37, African Development Bank, pp. 74-96.

Thomas, D. and J. Strauss (1997). "Health, wealth and wages of men and women in urban Brazil", *Labour and Population Working* paper 95, Vol. 11. Santa Monica CA: RAND, pp. 37-54.

15

Prevalence of Malnutrition among Male and Female of Annavaram Village, Visakhapatnam, Andhra Pradesh

Sagar Chettri

Introduction

When there is a lack of or excess intake of one or more nutrients and fatal utilization of nutrients in our body, it leads to a state of imbalance in the body. This condition is known as malnutrition. Malnutrition can be defined as the insufficient, excessive or imbalanced consumption of nutrients. It refers to both under-nutrition and over-nutrition. In both the cases, it has a negative impact on the normal functioning of the body. Due to poor nutrition, the normal growth process and functioning slows down, thus leading to small adult body size. As a result of insufficient and inadequate amount of proteins and calories in the diet, a number of nutritional problems collectively known as protein-calorie malnutrition are caused (Releford, 2010). According to the World Health Organization, malnutrition is the most common nutritional disorder of the world (WHO, 1998). Recent research in the field of health in India has drawn attention to double burden of malnutrition, which is the co-existence of a high prevalence of underweight and a rising prevalence of obesity (Griffiths and Bentley, 2001).

Obesity is defined as a disease in which excess body fat has accumulated to an extent that health is adversely affected (WHO, 1998). It increases the chances of a person falling prey to the other non-communicable diseases and has become the sign of the changing face of malnutrition in developing countries (Ellulu *et al.,* 2014). If an individual has a BMI from 25-29.9 kg/m^2, he or she is considered as overweight. Having a BMI greater than or equal to 30 kg/m^2 is considered as obese (WHO, 2000). The risks of chronic diseases have increased as BMI has escalated resulting in obesity. These diseases include cardiovascular diseases, diabetes, musculoskeletal disorders, cancer, and premature death. Changes in dietary and physical activity patterns are often the result of environmental and societal changes associated with development and lack of supportive policies in sectors such as health, agriculture, transport, urban planning, environment, food processing, distribution, marketing and education (Ellulu *et al.*, 2014).

Malnutrition is a devastating problem, especially for people from low socio-economic status. Various socio-economic variables such as income, education, marital status, physical activity, occupation, and family type have an influence on the nutritional status of any individual. Therefore, present study focuses on the relationship of nutritional status and socio-economic conditions and lifestyles of males and females of Annavaram village.

It was found that the effect of parental economic status on over-weight among their children was slightly greater for those whose parental economic status were lower. It was also found that the effect of parental economic status on under-weight in their children slightly increased at lower levels of parental economic status (Noh *et al.* 2014). The population of both developed and developing countries is facing rapid increases in over-weight and obesity among children and adolescents. This is due to rapid socio-economic development, increasing sedentary lifestyle. The pattern of overweight and obesity differ by age, sex, socio-economic condition and rural-urban residence (Matijaasevich *et al.,* 2009). Study among the Meitei adolescent of Manipur, India also shows increase in the prevalence of overweight and obesity among the adolescents due to changes in dietary intake and an increasingly sedentary lifestyle (Singh and Dkhar, 2013). Study carried out by Kusuma and his colleagues from Andhra University in Visakhapatnam among two ethnic groups from each area type, namely, tribal, rural and urban areas, and samples of 646 men and 670 women belonging to six groups were selected on a multistage basis. Based on the measurements, the BMI was calculated. A considerable proportion of populations studied showed chronic energy deficiency (CED). A higher proportion of women than men showed CED (Kusuma *et al.*, 2008).

Objectives of the Present Study

1. To assess the nutritional status of male and female of Annavaram village of Andhra Pradesh.
2. To find the relationship between nutritional status and the socio-economic condition.

Materials and Methods

Period and Duration of Fieldwork

The present fieldwork study was conducted in Annavaram village from 17th December, 2015 to 5th January, 2016. No statistical sampling technique was applied in the selection of individual and household for the present study. I managed to collect data from 65 males and 91 females by survey of house to house visit.

Andhra Pradesh is located in the South-eastern coast of India. It is the eighth largest state of India with an area of 1,60,205 square kilometres. It is ranked tenth in terms of population with 4,93,86,799 people as per Census of India, 2011. In 2014, the north-western portion of the state was bifurcated and a new state of Telangana was formed. The state has a coastline of 974 km, the second longest among the states of India after Gujarat. It is bordered by Telangana in the north-west, Chhattisgarh in the north, Odisha in the north-east, Karnataka in the west, Tamil Nadu in the south and the water body of Bay of Bengal in the east.

Annavaram village is located 15 km east of Tagarapuvalasa, a town of Bheembli Mandal of Visakhapatnam district. This village lies between 17°30' N and 17°45' N latitude, and 83°15' E and 83°20' E longitude in the north coastal part of Andhra Pradesh. The entire village comprises Vada/Vodabalija caste, which is a traditional marine fishing community.

Anthropometry

The present study was conducted among the males and females

residing in the Annavaram village. Cross-sectional data on 65 males and 91 females aged between 5 and 75 years was collected for the present study. The data was collected through random sampling method following a survey of house to house visit. The subjects were divided as children (5–12 years), adolescents (13–19 years) and adults (20+ years). An anthropometric rod and a weighing scale to the nearest of 0.1 cm and 0.5 kg was used to measure the height and weight of the subjects wearing light clothes.

Data on Socio-Economic Conditions

Data on household income was collected directly from the subjects or the heads of the households. The incomes were cross-checked against certain aspects of socio-economic conditions like housing conditions, types of occupation, land holding and monthly expenditure. The per capita monthly income of the households was classified as follows:

Above 75th percentile (>Rs.2500) = High income group (HIG)

50th to 75th percentile (Rs.1500—Rs.2500) = Middle income group (MIG)

Below 50th percentile (< Rs.1500) = Low income group (LIG)

Data on educational attainment of individuals were classified into three categories, namely illiterate, primary and secondary and above. The primary level of education includes those individuals who studied up to V. In the secondary and above level of education, we included those who attended standard VI and above. Data on occupation of each subject were classified as students, fishermen, housewives, private and labourers.

Statistical Analysis

The data were analysed using MS-Excel software for the present research. The parameters taken were analyzed statistically to find out the mean, standard deviation for the anthropometric measurements. Prevalence of underweight, overweight and obesity has been evaluated using WHO standard value for adult males and females (WHO, 2000). According to it, BMI ≥ 30 kg/m² has been considered as obese, BMI between 25.0-29.9 kg/m² considered as overweight, BMI between 18.5-24.9 kg/m² is considered as normal and BMI below 18.5 kg/m² considered as underweight. The prevalence of underweight, overweight and obesity for children and adolescent has been classified by using z-scores for BMI for age and sex (WHO, 2007). According to the classification, BMI z-score >+2SD is considered as obese, BMI z-score >+1SD considered as overweight, BMI z-score between <–2SD and >+1SD is normal and BMI z-score < –2SD is considered as underweight. Prevalence of overweight/obesity was calculated in relation to different socio-economic conditions. In order to test the level of significance, t-test, ANOVA and chi-square have been used in the present study.

Results

Table 15.1 shows the nutritional status among children, adolescents and adults in males and females of Annavaram village. Table shows that the frequency of overweight/obese was higher among adult males (17.4%) and females (26.8%). In males, the frequency of overweight/obese (4.3%) was found in children. The frequency of underweight was found to be higher among the adolescent males (21.1%) followed by children (13.1%) and adult male (8.7%). Among female, the frequency of underweight was found higher in children (54.5%) followed by adolescent (35.7%) and adult (12.2%). The distribution of different BMI values in females was statistically significant (χ^2 = 23.42; df = 4; p<0.05).

The distribution of BMI values in relation with income among the males and females is shown in Table 15.2. The higher frequency of overweight/obese was found among the high income group in males (11.1%) and female (30.0%). This was followed by frequency of overweight/obese among the middle income group (7.7%) and lower income group (5.9%) in males. Among the females, the frequency of overweight/obese among the lower income group (12.8%) and middle income group (7.1%) was also found.

The frequencies of underweight 22.2 per cent, 15.4 per cent and 5.9 per cent was found among the high income, middle income and lower income respectively among the males. While the frequencies of underweight 20.0 per cent, 31.0 per cent and 30.8 per cent among

Table 15.1: Distribution of Different BMI Values among Males and Females of Annavaram Village

Age group	Number	Underweight	Normal	Over weight/Obese
MALE				
5—12	23	3 (13.1%)	19 (82.6%)	1 (4.3%)
13—19	19	4 (21.1%)	15 (78.9%)	0 (0.0%)
20+	23	2 (8.7%)	17 (73.9%)	4 (17.4%)
$\chi^2 = 5.884$; df = 4; p>0.05				
FEMALE				
5—12	22	12 (54.5%)	10 (45.5%)	0 (0.0%)
13—19	28	10 (35.7%)	18 (64.3%)	0 (0.0%)
20+	41	5 (12.2%)	25 (61.0%)	11 (26.8%)
$\chi^2 = 23.41$; df = 4; p <0.05				

Source: Master's Fieldwork.

Table 15.2: Distribution of Different BMI Value in Relation with Income among Males and Females of Annavaram Village

Income Group	Number	Underweight	Normal	Overweight/Obese
MALE				
Lower income	17	1 (5.9%)	15 (88.2%)	1 (5.9%)
Middle Income	39	6 (15.4%)	30 (76.9%)	3 (7.7%)
High Income	9	2 (22.2%)	6 (66.7%)	1 (11.1%)
$\chi^2 = 1.88$; df = 4; p>0.05				
FEMALE				
Lower income	39	12 (30.8%)	22 (56.4%)	5 (12.8%)
Middle Income	42	13 (31.0%)	26 (61.9%)	3 (7.1%)
High Income	10	2 (20.0%)	5 (50.0%)	3 (30.0%)
$\chi^2 = 4.11$; df = 4; p>0.05				

Source: Master's Fieldwork.

female was found in the high income, middle income and low income groups respectively. In case of males, the differences in the distribution of different BMI values in different income groups were not statistically significant ($\chi^2 = 1.88$; df = 4; p>0.05). Similarly, in females, the differences in the distribution of different BMI values in different income groups were not statistically significant ($\chi^2 = 4.11$; df = 4; p>0.05).

The distribution of overweight/obese and underweight in relation with educational level among males and females of Annavaram village is given in Table 15.3. The Table shows that the frequency of overweight/obese was higher among primary level of education in males (13.1%) and it was found higher among the illiterate in females (26.1%). Among the males, the frequency of overweight/obese of 3.1 percent was found among secondary and above level of education and 10.0 per cent among the illiterates. While in females, the frequency of overweight/obese was found to be 16.6 per cent in primary level of education.

Table 15.3: Distribution of BMI Values in Relation with Educational Level among Males and Females of Annavaram Village

Category	*Number*	*Underweight*	*Normal*	*Overweight/Obese*
MALE				
Illiterate	10	1 (10.0%)	8 (80.0%)	1 (10.0%)
Primary	23	3 (13.0%)	17 (73.9%)	3 (13.1%)
Secondary+	32	5 (15.6%)	26 (81.3%)	1 (3.1%)
$\chi^2 = 2.08$; df = 4; $p>0.05$				
FEMALE				
Illiterate	23	4 (17.4%)	13 (56.5%)	6 (26.1%)
Primary	30	8 (26.7%)	17 (56.7%)	5 (16.6%)
Secondary+	38	15 (39.5%)	23 (60.5%)	0 (0.0%)
$\chi^2 = 11.39$; df = 4; $p <0.05$				

Source: Master's Fieldwork.

Table 15.3 also shows that the frequency of underweight in males among the illiterate, primary and secondary and above level of education was 10.0 per cent, 13.0 per cent and 15.6 per cent respectively. In females, the frequency was 10.0 per cent, 13.1 per cent and 13.1 per cent among the illiterate, primary and secondary and above level of education respectively.

In males, the differences in the distribution of different BMI values in different educational levels were not statistically significant (χ^2 = 2.08; df = 4; $p>0.05$). In females, the differences in the distribution of different BMI values in different educational levels were statistically insignificant (χ^2 = 11.39; df4; $p <0.05$).

The distribution of BMI values in relation with occupation among males is shown in Table 15.4. Table shows that the higher frequency of overweight/obese (20.0%) was found among the private employees

Table 15.4: Distribution of BMI Values in Relation with Occupation among Males of Annavaram Village

Category	*Number*	*Under weight*	*Normal*	*Overweight/Obese*
MALE				
Student	42	7 (16.7%)	34 (80.9%)	1 (2.4%)
Fishermen	18	1 (5.6%)	14 (77.8%)	3 (16.6%)
Private and Labourer	5	1 (20.0%)	3 (60.0%)	1 (20.0%)

$\chi^2 = 5.93$; df = 4; $p>0.05$
Source: Master's Fieldwork.

and labourers. This was followed by frequency of overweight/obese among the fishermen (16.6%) and students (2.4%). The frequency of underweight among the private employees and labourers was the highest (20.0%). This was followed by frequency of underweight among the students (16.7%) and the fishermen (5.6%). The differences in the distribution of different BMI values in different occupations were not statistically significant ($\chi^2 = 5.93$; df = 4; $p>0.05$).

The distribution of BMI values in relation with occupation among the females is shown in Table 15.5. This Table shows that the higher frequency of overweight/obese was found among the housewife (30.6%). The frequency of underweight among the others (55.6%) was the highest, which was followed by the students (41.3%) and housewife (8.3%).

Table 15.5: Distribution of BMI Values in Relation with Occupation among Females of Annavaram Village

Category	*Number*	*Under weight*	*Normal*	*Overweight/Obese*
FEMALE				
Student	46	19 (41.3%)	27 (58.7%)	0 (0.0%)
Housewife	36	3 (8.3%)	22 (61.1%)	11 (30.6%)
Others	9	5 (55.6%)	4 (44.4%)	0 (0.0%)

$\chi^2 = 26.81$; df = 4; $p<0.05$
Source: Master's Fieldwork.

Discussion

The present research shows the nutritional status of the males and females in the village of Annavaram, Andhra Pradesh. The distribution of underweight and overweight/obese in relation with various socio-economic conditions such as income, education, dietary habits and leisure activities are discussed in the present study. The study shows that the frequency of underweight is higher among the children in both males and females. Children are most vulnerable to malnutrition due to low dietary intakes, inequitable distribution of food within the household, improper food storage and preparation, infectious disease and care (Grima and Genebo, 2002). The studies also indicate that the adult males and adult females show higher frequency of overweight/obese.

Economic status is an important factor explaining the nutritional status of an individual. On comparison with those with higher income, those with lower income were more likely to be under-nourished (Grima and Genebo, 2002). Among the children, adolescent and adult males, the prevalence of overweight/obese and underweight shows fluctuations in the present study. The frequency of overweight/obese in males, however, increases with increasing income level of the family. Similarly in females, higher frequency of overweight/obese is found among the higher income group.

The study shows fluctuations in the prevalence of overweight/obese and underweight in relation with education level among males. However, among the females, there is an increase in the frequency of underweight with increasing levels of education and decrease in the frequency of overweight with increasing level of education. The education level of people was low and majority of the people categorized under secondary and above included those people who had just passed the eighth standard or matriculation. As a result of this the awareness and knowledge about proper nutrition and health care are very less. Among the males, the prevalence of underweight is higher among the private employees and labourers than the fishermen. Compared to the fishermen who had more amount of leisure time, the working hours of the private employees and labourers are greater resulting in greater frequency of underweight in them. Among the females, the frequency of underweight is higher among those working as labourers and private employees as well.

The present study mainly focuses on the distribution of BMI values and its relation with various socio-economic conditions prevalent. Compared with similar studies, the prevalence of under-nourished population was found to be higher among the studied community. The time period of the fieldwork being very limited, and also most of the adolescent boys being out of village for jobs, the sample size is less in my present study. But even then, I believe that this study will put forward among the people, the prevalence of malnutrition and obesity among the people of the small fishing community. It can be used to create awareness among the people regarding the importance of health, and the impact that various socio-economic factors have on the well-being of the people.

Conclusion

The present study shows the distribution of different BMI values among the male and female of Annavaram village in relation with different socio-economic conditions. The study shows that the prevalence of underweight and overweight/obesity is greatly influenced by certain socio-economic factors like family income, education, and occupation.

Acknowledgements

Author like to express his sincere gratitude to Dr. Maibam Samson Singh and Dr. K.R. Rama Mohan, for their help and support and Research participants for their co-operation during the fieldwork.

References

Dipietro, J.A., Costigan, K.A., Hilton, S.C., Pressman, E.K. (1999). "Effects of socio-economic status and psychological stress on the development of the fetus", *NY Academy of Science,* 49: 356-58.

Ellulu, M., Abed, Y., Rahmat, A., Ranneh, Y. and Ali, F. (2014). "Epidemiology of obesity in developing countries: Challenges and prevention", *Glob EpidemiObes.*, 2:2.

Griffiths, P.L., Bentley, M.E. (2001). "The nutrition transition is underway in India", *J Nutr.,* 131: 2692-2700.

Kusuma, Y.S. and Das, P.K. (2008). "Hypertension in Orissa, India: A cross-sectional study among some tribal, rural and urban population", *Public Health*, 122:1120-1123.

Matijasevich, A., Victoria, C.G., Golding, J., Barros, F.C., Menezes, A.M., Araujo, C.L., Smith, G.D. (2009). "Socio-economic position and overweight among adolescents: Data from birth cohert studies in Brazil and the UK, *BMC Pub. Hlth.,* 9: 105-112.

Naidu, N.A., Rao, P.N. (1994). "Body mass index: A measure of nutritional status in Indian population", *Eur. J. ClinNutr.*, 48:131-40.

Noh, J.W., Kim, Y., Park, J., Oh. I.W., Kwon, Y.D. (2014). "Impact of parental socio-economic status on childhood and adolescent overweight and underweight in Korea", *Journal of Epidemiology,* 24(3):221-229.

Ogden, L.C., Molly, M.L., Carroll, M.D., Flegal, K.M. (2010). "Obesity and socio-economic status in adults: United States, 2005-2008", *National Centre for Health Statistics,* 50:1-8.

Releford, J. (2010). *The Human Species: An Introduction to Biological Anthropology*, 8th ed., New York: McGraw

Shetty, P.S. (1984). "Adaptive changes in basal metabolic rate and lean body mass in chronic undernutrition", *Hum. Nutr.Clin.*, 38: 443-451.

Singh, M.S. and Dkhar, J.W. (2013). "Growing obese in Manipur: Relationship between age and obesity among the Meitei males of Manipur, India", *Anthropologist,* 16(3): 753-756.

UNICEF (1990). *Strategy for Improved Nutrition of Children and Women in Developing Countries*, New York: UNICEF.

WHO (1998). *Obesity: Preventing and Managing the Global Epidemic*, Report of a WHO Consultation on Obesity, Geneva: World Health Organisation.

WHO (2000). *The Asia-Pacific Perspective: Redefining Obesity and its Treatment*, Melbourne: Health Communications, Australia.

Index

CPC 1/24